"The feet speak what the lips cannot."

— Ancient Proverb

Signs and Meanings:

What the Feet Reveal About Health, Stress, and the Body's Story

This book is a companion to *Secrets of a Healer: Magic of Reflexology*, offering deeper insights into the visual and tactile signs found on the feet and what they may reveal about a person's health and well-being.

Dr. Constance Santego
Maximillian Enterprises
Kelowna, BC

Copy Editor and Interior Design: Constance Santego
Book Layout: ©2017 BookDesignTemplates.com

Ordering Information:
Quantity sales. Special discounts are available on quantity purchases by corporations, associations, and others. For details, contact the "Special Sales Department" at the address above.

Trade paperback ISBN: 978-1-990062-67-4
eBook ISBN 978-1-990062-68-1

Created and published In Canada. Printed and bound in the United States of America

Published by Maximillian Enterprises
Kelowna, BC
Canada
www.maximilliane.com

Dedication

To my first Reflexology teacher,
Diane Wiebe

Your guidance opened my eyes—
not just to the feet, but to the stories they hold.
From that first moment we met, you saw something in me I
hadn't yet seen in myself.
This book is a reflection of the journey you set in motion, and
the thousands of steps that followed.

Thank you for being the spark.
You are, and always will be, a true Earth Angel.

ALSO BY DR. CONSTANCE SANTEGO

NOVELS

Illegitimate Grace

Okanagan Trilogy:
Beneath the Vineyards
Under the Okanagan Sun
Guardian of the Lake

The Nine Spiritual Gifts Series:
Journey of a Soul – (Vol 1 Michael)
Language of a Soul – (Vol 2 Gabriel)
Prophecy of a Soul – (Vol 3 Bath Kol)
Healing of a Soul – (Vol 4 Raphael)
Miracles of a Soul – (Vol 5 Hamied)
Knowledge of a Soul – (Vol 6 Raziel)
Wisdom of a Soul – (Vol 7 Uriel)
Faith of a Soul – (Vol 8 Pistis Sophia)

NONFICTION

The Intuitive Life, The Gift Of Prophecy, Third Edition
Fairy Tales, Dreams And Reality… *Where Are You On Your Path?*
Second Edition
Your Persona… The Mask You Wear
Archangel Michael's Soul Retrieval Guide
Tesla And The Future Of Energy Medicine
Beyond Tesla: *Advancing The Science Of Energy Healing*
Tesla's Code: *Mastering Energy, Frequency, And Creative Power*
Scaling Beyond 6 Figures: *Strategies for Health & Wellness Professionals*
Beyond the Mind: *Harnessing the Power of Astral Projection for Creative Awakening*
Bend, Don't Break: *Finding Your Way Back to Abundance*
Ring Therapy: *A Guide to Healing and Balance*
Ring Therapy Pocket Guide
Floraopathy™: The Art and Science of Vibrational Healing with Essential Oils

REIKI WISDOM, SERIES:

Angelic Lifestyle, a Vibrant Lifestyle
Angelic Lifestyle 42-Day Energy Cleanse
Reiki and the Power of The Joint Points: *Unlocking Energy Pathways for Healing* (Vol I)
Reiki and Karmic Healing: *Releasing Patterns From Past Lives* (Vol II)
Reiki And The Five Elements (Vol III)

SECRETS OF A HEALER, SERIES:
Magic Of Aromatherapy (Vol I)
Magic Of Reflexology (Vol II)
Magic Of The Gifts (Vol III)
Magic Of Muscle Testing (Vol IV)
Magic Of Iridology (Vol V)
Magic Of Massage (Vol VI)
Magic Of Hypnotherapy (Vol VII)
Magic Of Reiki (Vol VIII)
Magic Of Advanced Aromatherapy (Vol IX)
Magic Of Esthetics (Vol X)
The Reiki Master's Manual (Vol XI)

ADULT COLORING JOURNALS

SERIES-ZEN COLORING:
Quantum Energy and Mindful Living Journal (Vol 1)
Reiki Energy Journal (Vol 2)
Nine Spiritual Gifts Journal (Vol 3)
I Forgive Journal (Vol 4)

FOR CHILDREN
I am Big Tonight. I Don't Need the Light

Contents

Preface

Since 1997, I've worked with thousands of feet—and each one has told a story.

At first glance, reflexology may seem like a technique: press here, relieve pain there. But for those of us who have practiced it long enough, a deeper truth emerges. The feet hold signs— visual, tactile, and energetic clues about what the body has endured, what it's experiencing now, and sometimes what it's still trying to process. These markings are not random. They're messages.

Over the years, I began to notice patterns. A red patch here, a hollow spot there. Puffy tissue in one area, rigid tension in another. I started asking my clients questions. What I heard in return—over and over again—was consistent. The stories behind their symptoms matched the areas where these signs appeared.

This book is a collection of what I've learned from listening to those feet.

Let me be clear: this isn't about guessing. It's not vague intuition. It's observation backed by repetition. When you hear the same answers to the same patterns across hundreds of people, you begin to understand that the feet carry a wisdom of their own. They reflect our stress, our injuries, our habits, and even our healing.

The signs I share with you in this book—puffiness, hollows, calluses, tightness, color changes, and more—are not just theory. They come from real client experiences, gathered over decades in practice. While I can't tell you the exact diagnosis or when a condition began, I can tell you what to look for, what it often means, and how to support the body in its healing process.

Signs and Meanings is a companion to my book *Secrets of a Healer: Magic of Reflexology*, and is intended to deepen your practice—whether you're a practitioner, a student, or simply someone curious about what your own feet might be trying to tell you.

The body speaks. The feet whisper.
Let's begin to listen—together.

Dr. Constance Santego Ph.D.
Doctor of Natural Medicine

Note to Reader

Reflexology is not a replacement for modern medicine. Your doctor remains a vital part of your healthcare team—and if I were to break my leg, I'd want every nurse, doctor, and hospital staff member available to help me heal.

But where modern medicine excels in crisis care, Eastern medicine offers something equally important: *balance.* In my experience, the Eastern approach teaches that we are active participants in our health—not passive recipients waiting for something to go wrong. It emphasizes prevention, stress reduction, vital energy flow, and conscious choices about what we put into both our bodies and our minds.

Reflexology is one of those tools. It's a hands-on technique, yes—but it's also a pathway. A bridge to the subconscious. A way to access the body's innate intelligence and healing potential.

When practiced with sensitivity, honesty, and integrity, reflexology becomes more than a method—it becomes a practice of self-awareness and self-care. It invites you to tune in. To pay attention. And to honor the quiet signs your body has been offering all along.

Shift happens… and with it, healing becomes possible. Create magic.

Learning Outcome

By the time you've completed this book and explored the signs, meanings, and techniques within, you will:

- Gain a foundational understanding of reflexology and how the feet reflect the body's systems.
- Learn techniques to stimulate homeostasis—encouraging the body's natural ability to balance and heal.
- Deepen your observational and intuitive skills to support healing on the physical, mental, emotional, and spiritual levels.

This book is both a practical guide and an invitation to expand your awareness—to see the feet not just as structure, but as story.

Limitations

Reflexology is a powerful and supportive therapy—but like all healing modalities, it has its limitations. While it can complement many conditions and support the body's healing processes, reflexology should not be considered a cure-all. In many cases, it works best as part of an integrated wellness plan, supporting—but not replacing—the primary care provided by physicians or specialized practitioners.

As a reflexologist, one of your most important responsibilities is knowing when to refer your client to another healthcare professional. Collaboration with other disciplines enhances the client's overall care and builds trust in your practice.

Ethical and Legal Limitations

Most of the limitations in reflexology relate not to what the therapy *can* do, but to what practitioners *are legally permitted* to say or do. Unless you hold a license as a medical doctor or regulated healthcare provider with diagnostic authority, there are certain actions you must not take:

1. You Cannot Diagnose

Only licensed physicians or regulated healthcare professionals with a provincially approved scope of practice may diagnose a condition.

Instead of saying,

"You have liver problems,"
a reflexologist should say,
"The liver reflex area feels tender today,"
or
"I'm noticing some sensitivity in this reflex zone."

If a client's reflex reaction causes concern, always recommend that they follow up with their physician or specialist.

2. You Cannot Prescribe

You may not advise clients to start, stop, or adjust any medications—including herbal, natural, or over-the-counter remedies.

If you want to share information, use phrases such as:

- "I've personally used ___ and found it helpful."
- "Some people have shared that ___ has supported them."
- "You may wish to speak to a qualified herbalist or naturopath about that."

3. You Cannot Treat a Specific Condition

Reflexologists do not work to resolve specific diagnosed conditions. Instead, we work the *entire body through the reflex zones*, supporting the body's natural healing and balance.

If you suspect an imbalance in a certain system, it is appropriate to revisit that reflex area during the session—but always continue to treat holistically, not symptomatically.

4. Use of Instruments

Some schools teach reflexology with tools or instruments, while others teach hands-only techniques. Both approaches can be effective when used ethically and skillfully. In my training programs, I focus on hands-only methods to develop practitioner sensitivity and intuitive connection—but the use of tools remains a personal or school-based decision, provided it stays within ethical and safety standards.

Reflexology empowers the body to heal itself, but practitioners must remain grounded in ethical practice, respectful of scope, and aware of their role as part of a broader system of care. Knowing your limitations doesn't reduce your effectiveness—it enhances your professionalism and protects both you and your clients.

Chapter 1: The Language of the Feet

In 1997, I began a journey that would change the way I understood the human body forever.

At first, reflexology was simply another tool in my growing practice—a fascinating blend of Eastern theory, zone therapy, and hands-on healing. I had studied natural medicine, massage, and energy work, and reflexology felt like the perfect bridge between structure and energy, anatomy and emotion.

But the turning point came when I began to notice something unexpected: the feet were speaking.

Not with words, of course, but with texture, tension, markings, and subtle shifts that showed up session after session. A red patch here, a hollow there. Bony pressure, tight muscles, puffy pads. I started to ask questions. And what my clients told me— over and over again—was that these "foot signs" were not random. They often mirrored real conditions, past injuries, emotional trauma, or hidden imbalances.

It wasn't intuition alone. It was *pattern recognition.*

Over time, I began documenting everything I noticed. I tracked signs. I correlated them with what clients told me. I compared notes across years of sessions. Slowly, a second map of the feet began to emerge—one that extended beyond traditional reflex points and zones. It revealed not just where to press, but *what the body might be trying to say.*

That's what this book is about.

It's a companion to my previous work, *Secrets of a Healer: Magic of Reflexology*, but where that book focuses on the method, this one focuses on the *messages.* The subtle, often-overlooked signs that show up in the skin, structure, and sensation of the feet—and what those signs may mean.

This is not a diagnostic manual. I do not claim to diagnose or cure. What I offer here is decades of observation, client feedback, and healing insights gathered in the treatment room. Whether you are a reflexologist, bodyworker, energy healer, or simply someone curious about what your own body is revealing, my hope is that this book opens a new level of awareness in your practice—and in yourself.

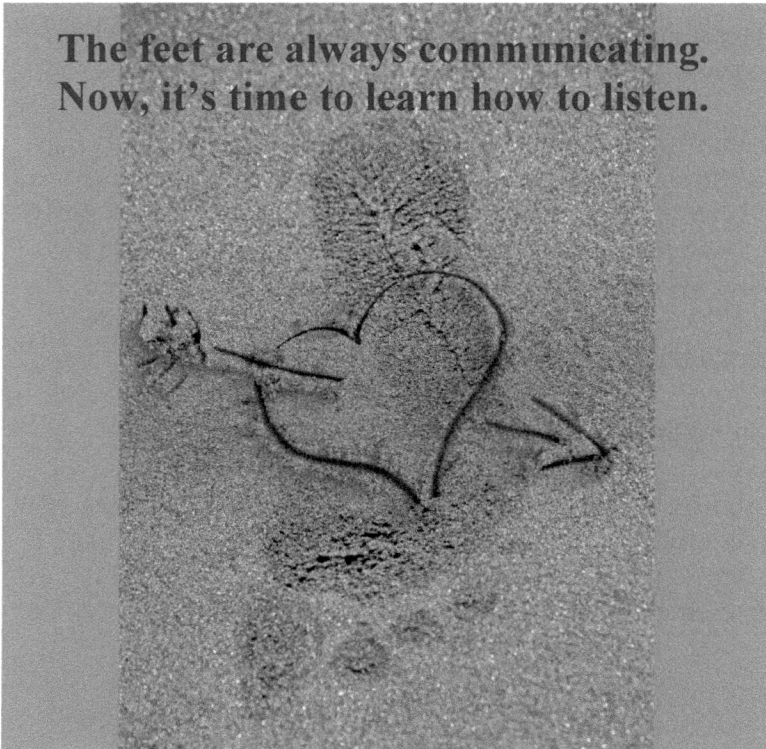

The feet are always communicating.
Now, it's time to learn how to listen.

Listening to the Body's Silent Signals

Not all pain speaks loudly.
Not all imbalances show up in bloodwork.
And not every client has the words—or even the awareness—to describe what's truly going on inside them.

That's where reflexology becomes something more than a technique. It becomes a way to *listen.*

The body speaks in subtle ways: through tension, through tightness, through shifts in temperature, texture, and tenderness. It whispers its warnings long before a crisis erupts. But we have to be trained not just to see and touch—but to interpret.

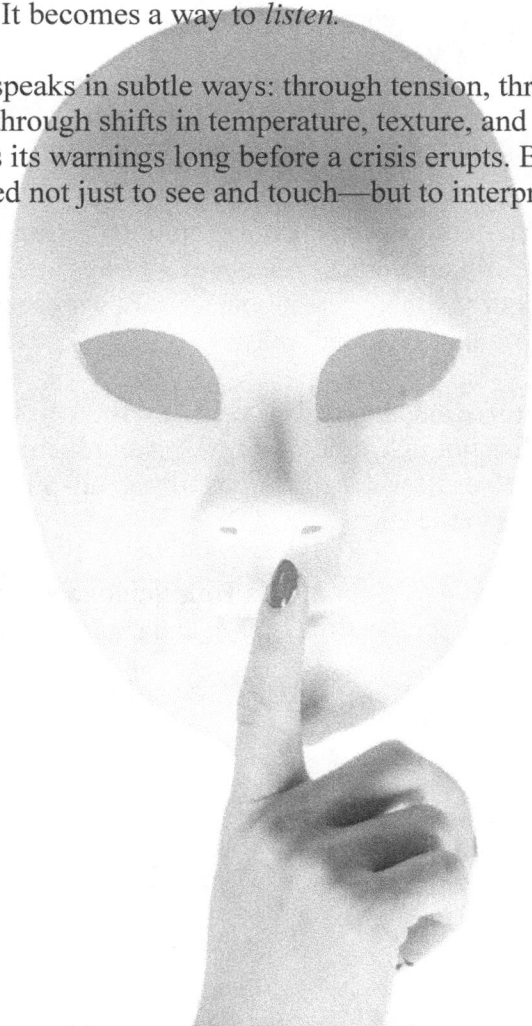

As reflexologists, we're often the ones who notice what others overlook. A slight puffiness near the sinus reflex, a gritty texture around the intestines, or a glowing white line beneath a toenail—all of these may offer clues the client hasn't yet connected. In many cases, they don't feel "sick," but something isn't quite right. Their body knows it. Their feet show it.

This is especially important for clients who:

- Are recovering from emotional trauma but can't verbalize it
- Have undiagnosed conditions still under investigation
- Feel disconnected from their physical body
- Are children, neurodivergent, or nonverbal
- Have long-standing tension patterns masked by coping mechanisms

In my practice, I've often found that clients begin to cry—not because of pain, but because they feel *seen*. Reflexology bypasses the defense systems and taps into something primal and receptive. When a practitioner gently brings attention to a certain reflex or texture, it creates space for awareness, healing, and often profound emotional release.

Listening to these silent signals is an act of respect. It reminds us that health is not just about fixing what's broken. It's about attuning ourselves to what's already shifting, adapting, and speaking beneath the surface.

This book, *Signs and Meanings*, is your guide to those signals—so you can see what others may miss, and offer support where it's needed most.

Observation vs. Assumption

In reflexology, as in all healing work, there is a fine line between observation and assumption.

Observation is grounded in experience. It is the act of noticing, without judgment, what is physically present. It's about gathering information—texture, temperature, puffiness, rigidity, color, shape—without jumping to conclusions. Observation keeps the practitioner in a state of curiosity. It allows space for discovery and invites dialogue between you and your client.

Assumption, on the other hand, is the act of assigning meaning without context or confirmation. It often stems from ego, fear, or the desire to have an answer before one is truly known. Assumptions can lead to misinformation, breach of trust, or even harm if a practitioner oversteps their role and speaks as if they know more than they do.

For example:

- Saying, "You have liver disease" is an assumption—and an unethical one.
- Saying, "The liver reflex feels tender today. Have you been feeling off lately?" is observation—and invites partnership.

A skilled reflexologist observes patterns over time. You may notice that many people with asthma have similar puffiness under the fifth toe, or that grief often shows up as tightness in the lung reflex. You might become familiar with the visual signs that show up in cases of IBS or gallbladder removal. These are valid patterns—but until your client confirms it, they remain *possibilities*, not *conclusions*.

In this book, I share what I've consistently observed in real clients over decades of practice. But even with strong patterns, I always encourage reflexologists to approach each session with humility, care, and respect for the unknown.

Your job is not to diagnose—it is to listen, support, and offer insight based on what you observe.

When you stay in the space of observation, not assumption, you become a trusted guide—not a guessing game.

How This Book Complements Secrets of a Healer: Magic of Reflexology

If you've read *Secrets of a Healer: Magic of Reflexology*, you've already explored the foundational techniques, zone theory, and intuitive tools of reflexology. That book was designed to teach **how to perform** reflexology—where to press, how to flow through a routine, and how to energetically tune in while working with the feet.

This book takes the next step.

Signs and Meanings focuses on **how to read** the feet—not just through reflex points, but through the **subtle signs and markings** that appear on the surface, in the tissue, and beneath your hands.

Where *Magic of Reflexology* teaches the art of activating healing through touch, this book teaches you to **see what the body is silently showing you** before you even begin your treatment.

Together, the two books form a complete experience:

- **One book shows you how to perform reflexology.**
- **The other shows you how to interpret what the feet reveal.**

They are two parts of the same journey—offering both practical technique and intuitive insight.

So whether you're a student, a seasoned practitioner, or someone simply curious about what your own feet are trying to say, this book was created to help you deepen your relationship with the wisdom beneath your soles.

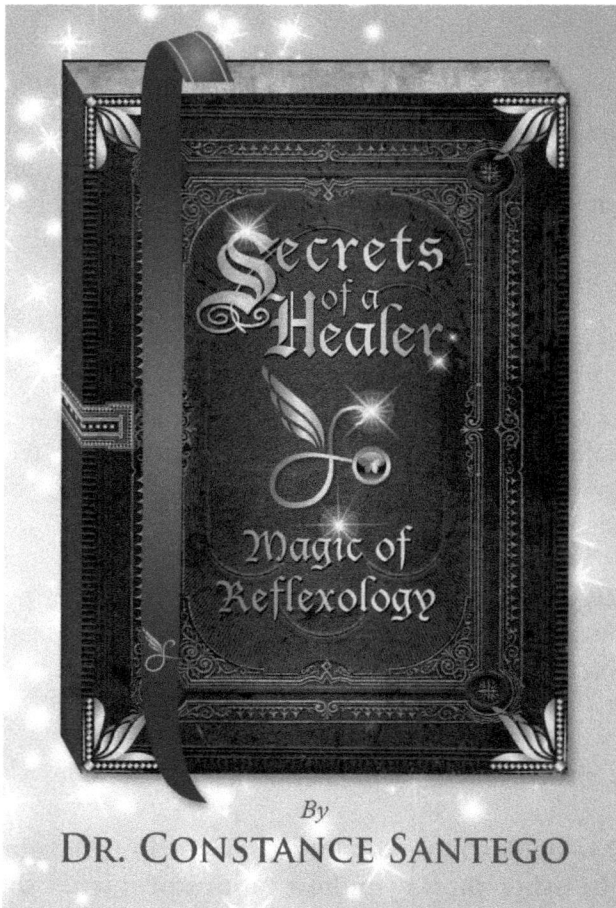

Chapter 2: The Basics of Reading Feet

Overview of Reflexology Zones and Organ System Connections

Reflexology is based on the principle that **the feet are a mirror of the entire body**. Every organ, gland, and system has a corresponding reflex point located on the soles, tops, sides, and even toes of the feet.

These points aren't randomly placed—they follow a **zone-based system** that gives structure and logic to the practice.

What Are Reflexology Zones?

The body is divided into **ten longitudinal zones**:

- **Five on the right side**, from the center of the body outward to the right shoulder and foot
- **Five on the left side**, mirroring the same from the center line to the left shoulder and foot

Each zone runs in a straight line from the **top of the head to the tips of the toes**, organizing the body and feet into matching vertical segments. If an organ or structure is located in a particular zone of the body, its reflex point will appear in the same zone of the foot.

For example:

- The **liver**, located on the right side of the body, is found only on the **right foot**
- The **heart**, slightly to the left of center in the chest, appears only on the **left foot**
- The **spine**, located at the centerline, runs down the **inner edge** of both feet

This structure, first popularized by Dr. William Fitzgerald as **Zone Therapy**, was later refined by Eunice Ingham into the reflexology charts we use today.

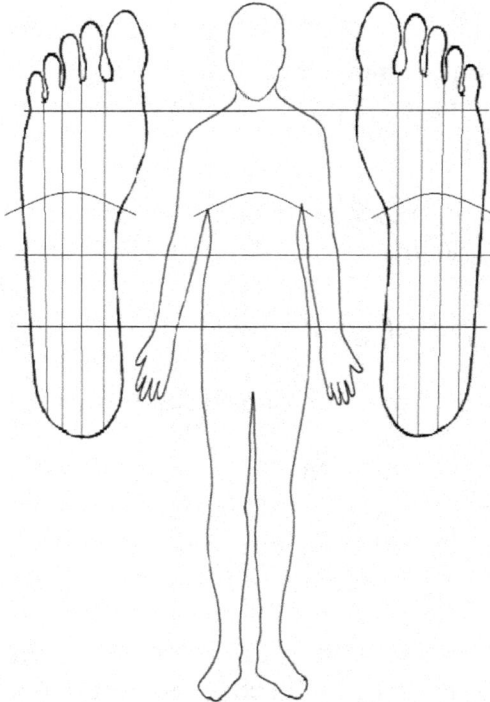

Major Reflex Zones and Their Organ Connections

Foot Region	Connected Body Systems/Organs
Toes	Head, brain, eyes, ears, sinuses, pituitary, pineal gland
Ball of the Foot	Lungs, heart, chest, shoulders, diaphragm
Arch (Midfoot)	Liver (right), stomach (left), pancreas, small intestines, kidneys
Heel	Colon, bladder, reproductive organs, sciatic nerve, hips, lower back
Inner Edge of Foot	Spine and central nervous system
Outer Edge of Foot	Arm, leg, lymph, gallbladder (right), spleen (left), knee, shoulder
Tips of Toes (Dorsal)	Teeth, dental work, stress in the jaw, brain congestion
Between Toes (Webbing)	Sinus drainage, lymphatic nodes, emotional sensitivity

Left Foot vs. Right Foot

Each foot not only reflects a side of the body—but also carries its own energetic signature:

- The **left foot** often reflects **feminine, emotional, internal** processes
- The **right foot** often reflects **masculine, logical, external** aspects

Some organs appear only on one side:

- **Left only:** Heart, spleen, descending colon
- **Right only:** Liver, gallbladder, ascending colon

Why the Zone System Matters

Understanding the zone system allows you to:

- Navigate the feet with clarity and confidence
- Correlate pain, tension, or signs in the feet to real-world concerns in the body
- Notice patterns that reflect physical, emotional, or energetic imbalances
- Avoid random treatment—your work becomes intentional, targeted, and effective

When used alongside the observational skills shared in this book—like interpreting puffiness, hollows, color changes, and more—the zone system becomes your **roadmap to the body's hidden messages**.

Key Indicators:

Texture, Color, Temperature, Shape, and Skin Markings

The surface of the foot is more than skin deep—it's a message board from the body, full of silent signals. As a reflexologist or intuitive practitioner, tuning in to **what you see, feel, and sense** is the foundation of effective reading. Each texture, tone, or temperature variation can offer clues about physical health, emotional patterns, or energy flow.

Let's break down the core indicators:

1. Texture

- **Dry, flaky skin**: Often suggests dehydration, poor circulation, or nutritional deficiencies. Emotionally, it may indicate detachment or lack of nourishment—physically or spiritually.
- **Rough patches or thickened skin**: May show long-standing stress or chronic tension in the corresponding reflex zone.
- **Gritty or sandy areas under the skin**: These may be felt during thumb walking and often suggest uric or lactic acid deposits. They indicate congestion or stagnation in that organ or system.
- **Spongey, soft, or mushy texture**: May suggest lymphatic issues, fluid retention, or fatigue in the area.
- **Hard, rigid skin**: May reflect long-term physical strain or hardened emotional patterns.

2. Color

The coloration of the feet gives real-time feedback about circulation, organ stress, and inflammation:

- **Redness**: Often shows inflammation or excess energy. Common over adrenal, lung, or joint reflexes.
- **Pallor or whiteness**: Can suggest poor circulation, depletion, or internal coldness.
- **Bluish tones**: May be a sign of stagnation, oxygen deprivation, or suppressed emotions.
- **Yellow tint**: May relate to liver or gallbladder stress, or detox pathways needing support.
- **Dark spots or discoloration**: May reflect trauma, stuck energy, or emotional memory held in the reflex area.

Note: Always assess color in context—temperature and lighting can affect how skin tones appear.

3. Temperature

- **Cold feet**: Often a circulatory concern, but can also show fear, adrenal fatigue, or disconnection from grounded energy.
- **Hot spots**: May reveal inflammation, infection, or overactive systems (i.e., liver, sinuses, or reproductive reflexes).
- **Temperature imbalance between feet or zones**: When one foot or area is consistently warmer or colder than its counterpart, it may highlight imbalance or compensation.

4. Shape

The structural shape of the foot tells a longer story—how the body has adapted over time:

- **Flat feet**: May relate to postural imbalances or energetic collapse (a lack of inner support).
- **High arches**: Sometimes linked with tight control, anxiety, or an overly rigid system.
- **Bulges or protrusions**: May indicate chronic inflammation or physical misalignment affecting the related zone.
- **Shortened toes or pulled-under toes**: Often reflect tension patterns, particularly in the spine or emotional system.
- **Wide forefoot vs. narrow heel**: This can suggest stress carried in the chest/lung area or balance issues between emotional expression and grounding.

5. Skin Markings

These include lines, calluses, scars, and discolorations that are especially significant in reading feet:

- **Calluses**: Often form where energy is chronically stuck. A hardened message—look at the reflex beneath for long-standing tension or unspoken emotional burden.
- **Horizontal lines**: May indicate life stages, stress phases, or energetic "breaks" from the past.
- **Cracks**: Often appear on dry heels or in the arch and may relate to emotional vulnerability or disconnection in the corresponding zone.
- **Moles or pigmentation**: Can signify energetic "hot spots" or inherited tendencies.

- **Scars**: Always ask where and how they formed—they may hold trauma, even if the physical healing is complete.

A Note for Practitioners

These indicators are not for diagnosis, but for **deeper inquiry**. A red patch or bony structure may point toward a trend, not a final answer. Your role is to **notice, ask gently**, and support the body's journey back to balance. When combined with reflex work, intuition, and ethical care, these signs become part of a larger healing map—one the feet are eager to share.

How to Assess with Neutrality and Curiosity — Not Fear or Prediction

The feet may show us many things—but what we *do* with that information matters most.

As reflexologists, we walk a fine line. On one side is insight. On the other, assumption. While the signs we observe—texture, temperature, shape, markings—can reveal profound truths, they must always be approached with **neutrality**, **curiosity**, and **respect** for the client's journey.

This means we:

- **Observe without judgment.** We note what we see and feel, but we don't label it as good or bad.
- **Ask without leading.** We may invite reflection—"Do you notice anything unusual in your digestion lately?"— but we never suggest a diagnosis.
- **Stay open to confirmation.** Our insights are valuable, but the client's experience must lead the conversation. They are the expert on their own body.
- **Hold space for mystery.** Not every sign has an immediate answer. Sometimes the body speaks in layers, and meaning becomes clearer over time.

Avoid fear-based language. It can do more harm than good. Telling a client, "This could mean something serious," or "You may have a heart issue," can cause panic, unnecessary worry, or even mistrust. Reflexology is not about predicting illness—it's about promoting awareness, balance, and healing.

Instead, use language like:

- "This reflex feels tender—sometimes I see this when someone's been under stress."
- "There's a puffiness in this area that may relate to congestion. Have you noticed anything like that?"
- "This area is showing a lot of tension. It might be helpful to support it with relaxation, stretching, or massage."

Neutrality keeps us grounded. Curiosity keeps us learning. Together, they create a safe space where healing can happen—without pressure, fear, or ego.

As you explore the signs and meanings in the coming chapters, remember:

- You're not here to predict the future.
- You're here to *witness the present*—and gently support the body's wisdom as it unfolds.

Practitioner Responsibilities and Ethical Boundaries

As reflexology steps deeper into the world of signs and meanings, it's crucial to remember: with observation comes responsibility. The more attuned you become to the body's signals, the more care must be taken in how that information is handled. Whether you're a certified reflexologist, energy healer, or holistic practitioner, ethical boundaries are your safeguard—and your strength.

1. Do Not Diagnose

Even if signs on the feet appear consistent with a condition you've seen before, **you are not a medical doctor** (unless specifically licensed to be one). You **cannot name diseases** or offer clinical diagnoses.

Instead of saying: "This looks like liver disease."
Say: "The liver reflex is showing tenderness or a textural change. You may want to explore that further with your doctor."

2. Work the Whole Body

Never treat one area only—even if the signs appear to localize there. Reflexology is a **balancing modality**, not a treatment for a single condition. Signs in one area may be compensating for imbalances elsewhere.

3. Respect Client Readiness

Some clients are emotionally or psychologically unprepared to explore the deeper meaning behind what their feet reveal. Always **ask permission** before discussing potential insights. Respect when they say, "I just want to relax today."

Use phrases like:

- "Would you like to hear what I've noticed energetically?"
- "Sometimes certain signs correlate with deeper patterns—are you open to that?"

4. Never Lead or Project

Let the client interpret first. What you see is a possibility, not a verdict. Offering a specific meaning too soon can unintentionally create fear or false belief.

Good practice: Ask, "Does that area feel familiar to you in any way?"

Poor practice: "This is where people hold cancer."

5. Honor Confidentiality

Everything a client shares—verbally or physically—must remain private. The stories told through their feet, markings, or emotional reactions are sacred. Even when sharing anonymized case studies, ensure details cannot identify a person.

6. Acknowledge Your Scope

Stay within your professional boundaries. You may recommend a client see their doctor, try massage, or consider emotional support, but **do not prescribe** supplements, treatments, or give medical opinions unless licensed to do so.

Instead, say:

- "Some clients have found chiropractic helpful with this area."
- "You might want to explore this with a naturopath or counselor."

7. Maintain a Neutral, Safe Presence

Your role is not to fix or label—it's to witness, support, and offer tools that assist the body in healing itself. The client's path is their own. Create a space free from judgment, fear-based language, or personal bias.

Your Responsibility Is Your Power

The deeper you read, the more trust you must hold. This is what separates a gifted practitioner from a careless one. When you pair insight with compassion and boundaries, your presence becomes healing—long before you even touch their feet.

Chapter 3: Feet Overall – The Whole-Foot Story

What the Feet Reveal Before Reflexology Begins

Before your hands ever make contact with the feet, the body is already speaking.

Reflexology is more than a method—it's a dialogue. And that dialogue starts the moment a client removes their socks. Often, the feet present signs and sensations that offer a prelude to the session's deeper work. These subtle cues can tell you volumes about the client's physical, emotional, and energetic state— **before a single reflex is activated.**

1. Posture and Tension

How a client **places or holds their feet** when they sit or recline can be revealing:

- Are the feet turned inward or outward?
- Do the ankles cross protectively?
- Is one foot stiff while the other relaxes?

These positions may hint at discomfort, guarded emotions, or habitual compensation patterns within the musculoskeletal system.

2. Skin Texture and Tone

Even without touch, you can visually note:

- **Dry or cracked heels** – often associated with adrenal fatigue or emotional rigidity.
- **Pale feet** – may suggest poor circulation or energetic depletion.
- **Redness** – can indicate inflammation or overactivity.
- **Calluses and corns** – mark areas of long-term stress or protection.

3. Swelling or Puffiness

Swelling often reflects lymphatic stagnation, water retention, or unresolved grief. The top of the foot may indicate fluid in the upper body (sinuses, lungs), while puffiness near the ankles could relate to kidney, reproductive, or circulatory strain.

4. Toenails and Nail Beds

Toenails may show nutritional deficiencies, fungal issues, or trauma history:

- **Thickened or yellow nails** – often fungal, but may also indicate suppressed detox pathways.
- **Ridges or spooning** – can reflect stress, iron imbalance, or long-term tension.
- **Biting or picking at toes/nails** – unconscious self-soothing or anxiety patterns.

5. Odor and Temperature

- **Cold feet** may indicate thyroid concerns, circulation issues, or an emotional shutdown.
- **Excessive heat** can be linked to inflammation or agitation.
- **Odor** may suggest systemic imbalance, poor digestion, or elimination overload.

Note: Never shame or comment on these observations directly. If there is strong odor or visible signs of infection, approach with professionalism and care, and consider a referral if needed.

6. Foot Shape and Structure

Observe the arch, heel width, and toe position:

- **Flat feet** may indicate kidney imbalance, lack of grounding, or physical fatigue.
- **High arches** are often tied to anxiety or stored tension.
- **Bunions and toe overlaps** may reflect long-term joint stress, imbalance, or suppressed emotional expression.

7. Emotional Energy

Some clients' feet visibly "pull back" from being seen. This can present as:

- Flinching, curling toes, or sudden chill
- Covering one foot while exposing the other
- Apologizing for their feet's appearance

These subtle gestures may indicate **emotional vulnerability**, shame, or resistance to receiving care. Your calm, accepting presence makes all the difference.

Start Listening Before You Touch

As you prepare for a session, take a quiet moment to observe. The feet are already sharing insights. They may whisper stories of stress, reveal areas that crave attention, or uncover long-held emotions.

The art of reflexology begins in stillness. And in that stillness, the feet begin to speak.

Assessing Skin, Nails, Hydration, Circulation, and Odor

Before applying any reflexology techniques, your first role as a practitioner is to observe—with discernment, not judgment. The surface of the feet can reveal deep internal patterns. A skilled reflexologist learns to assess outer signs as indicators of the body's overall wellness, hydration levels, organ function, and emotional tone.

1. Skin: Texture, Thickness, and Integrity

The skin of the feet acts like a map—offering insight into physical and energetic states.

- **Dry, cracked skin** (especially on heels) often indicates dehydration, adrenal stress, or emotional hardness.
- **Excessively moist skin** may suggest a sluggish lymphatic system or hormonal imbalances.
- **Peeling skin** between toes might signal fungal infections or unresolved emotional irritability.
- **Calluses or corns** form in areas where pressure has built up over time—physically, emotionally, or posturally.

Practitioner Tip: Run your fingers gently over the skin's surface. Use clean fingertips (never fingernails) to detect areas of sandiness, grit, or soft swelling.

2. Nails: Clues to Nutrient Absorption and Stress

Toenails offer important clues regarding systemic health.

- **Brittle or splitting nails** may indicate poor nutrient absorption (particularly protein, biotin, or essential fatty acids).
- **White spots** are often associated with zinc deficiency or past trauma to the nail matrix.
- **Thickened or yellow nails** could be fungal, but might also reflect stagnation in the detoxification pathways or respiratory system.
- **Ridges (vertical or horizontal)** may point to long-term stress, thyroid imbalance, digestion issues, or past trauma (horizontal—from nail bed, every 1/8" is a month ago).

Observation Only: Reflexologists do not trim or treat nails. Refer to a podiatrist if the nail condition appears medical in nature.

3. Hydration

Hydration isn't just about how much water a person drinks—it's about how well their body retains and distributes fluids.

- **Tight, papery skin** often signals chronic dehydration.
- **Sunken areas** (especially at the tops of the feet) can suggest a lack of internal moisture.
- **Puffiness or edema** is commonly associated with water retention, poor kidney function, or congested lymph flow.

Hydration Check: Gently pinch a small area of the top of the foot. If the skin doesn't return quickly to shape, it may indicate dehydration.

4. Circulation

Circulatory health directly affects the color and temperature of the feet.

- **Cold feet** may be linked to anemia, hypothyroidism, or circulatory inefficiency.
- **Blue/purple undertones** could suggest oxygenation issues or venous insufficiency.
- **Redness or hot patches** are signs of inflammation, irritation, or overactive systems (like liver or adrenal strain).
- **Blanching (whiteness under pressure)** may indicate low blood pressure or poor peripheral circulation.

Simple Check: Press your thumb gently on the top of the foot for a few seconds and observe the refill time. Slow return of color may suggest compromised circulation.

5. Odor

Foot odor is not only about hygiene—it can point to internal imbalances.

- **Sweet, yeasty odor** might indicate candida or blood sugar irregularities.
- **Sharp or sour smell** may reflect liver overload or stress sweat (from adrenal surges).
- **Metallic or ammonia-like smell** can point to kidney strain or protein metabolism issues.

Respectful Practice: Never shame or comment directly on odor. Instead, consider it a clinical clue. Offer guidance only if invited or if a referral is warranted.

Putting It All Together

Use all your senses—sight, smell, touch, and intuition—to build a first impression of the client's internal state. This non-verbal dialogue can guide your session's focus and inform your questions, always delivered with care, neutrality, and compassion.

Foot Shape, Arch Height, Symmetry, and Postural Clues

The overall structure of the foot offers foundational insight into a client's physical alignment, stress distribution, and even emotional tendencies. Unlike isolated reflex points, these macro-level features speak to *how a person lives in their body*—how they carry their weight, process emotion, and adapt to chronic stress over time.

1. Foot Shape: The Foundation Blueprint

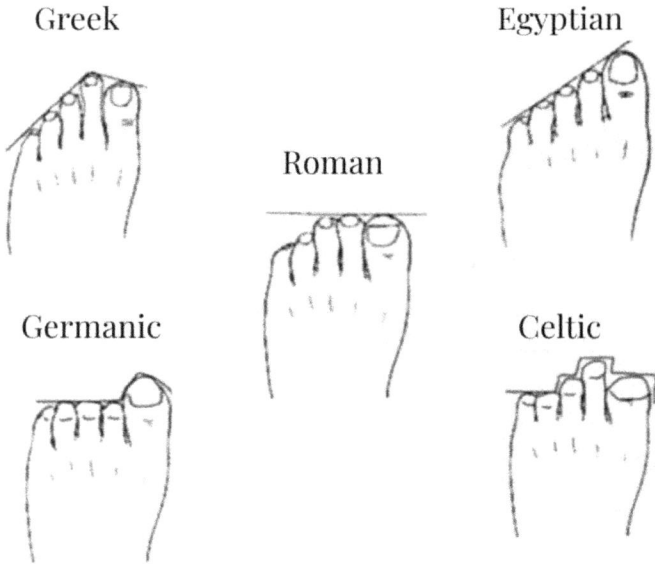

Greek

Egyptian

Roman

Germanic

Celtic

Foot shape varies widely from person to person and reflects both genetics and functional adaptation.

- **Square Foot (Peasant Foot)** – Toes are similar in length. Indicates steadiness, practicality, and resilience. Clients often have solid physical endurance but may experience issues in joints due to rigidity.
- **Greek Foot** – Second toe longer than the big toe. Often associated with leadership tendencies, drive, and a forward-thinking mind. Prone to postural imbalances and bunions.
- **Egyptian Foot** – Toes slope down gradually. Seen in flexible, sensitive types. Can reflect a more intuitive, emotionally attuned constitution. Watch for tight calves and lower back stress.

Tip: The shape of the foot often mirrors personality tendencies—groundedness, assertiveness, or sensitivity—and helps you customize pressure and approach.

Greek Foot Personality Tendencies

The **Greek foot shape**, also known as the **Flame Foot** or **Morton's Toe**, is identified by a **second toe that is longer than the big toe**, often with the remaining toes tapering down in length. This dynamic shape is packed with expressive energy—both physically and emotionally.

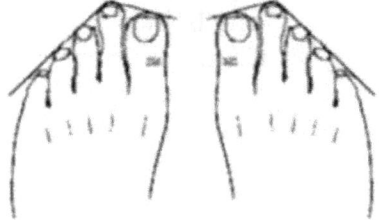

1. Energetic & Passionate

The extended second toe reflects **drive, enthusiasm, and a fiery spirit**. Greek-footed individuals are often **active, expressive, and full of creative energy**. They feel things deeply and tend to pour themselves into whatever they do.

2. Leaders & Motivators

This foot shape often appears in **natural motivators, teachers, coaches, and performers**. They have a talent for **rallying others**, sparking ideas, and pushing through obstacles. Their energy can be contagious—uplifting those around them.

3. Impulsive & Restless

While their passion is a gift, it can sometimes lead to **impatience or impulsive decisions**. They may struggle with burnout if they don't channel their energy constructively. They thrive with variety and movement but can become frustrated with routine or stagnation.

4. Strong-Willed & Opinionated

Greek-footed individuals **stand firm in their beliefs**. While not always confrontational, they are **assertive** and may have strong views on how things *should* be done. This confidence often earns them respect, though it may occasionally cause friction.

5. Creative & Visionary

Their energy isn't just physical—it's also highly creative. Greek-footed people often **think outside the box**, embrace the arts, or pursue innovation in their field. They're drawn to **inspiration, expression, and purpose**.

6. Emotionally Charged

Beneath the boldness is a deep emotional current. These individuals **feel intensely** and may need safe outlets to release stress or passion. They benefit from mindfulness and grounding practices to help **balance their fire with flow**.

Reflexology/Bodywork Tips for Greek Feet:

- **Pressure Preference:** Medium to firm pressure— especially along the second toe and ball of the foot (which may carry tension).
- **Best Techniques:** Deep tissue kneading, targeted pressure point work, and cooling or calming strokes to balance their high energy.
- **Connection Style:** Use inspiring language but offer structure—they appreciate encouragement *and* direction.
- **Healing Focus:** Grounding and calming therapies are key. Focus on balancing Solar Plexus and Heart Chakra energy to help align passion with peace.

Roman Foot Personality Tendencies

The **Roman foot shape**—also known as the **Square** or **Peasant** foot—is characterized by the first three toes being **almost the same length**, followed by the fourth and fifth descending in a more tapered slope. The overall appearance is broad and balanced, with a strong, square front.

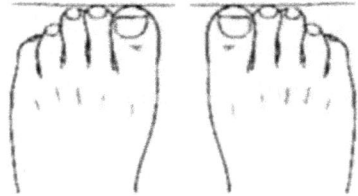

1. Grounded & Practical

People with Roman feet are **solid, dependable, and well-grounded**. They tend to be **realists** who deal with the world in a balanced and thoughtful way. Practicality is one of their strongest traits—they like to **understand how things work** before diving in.

2. Natural Leaders

This foot shape reflects a **natural leadership quality**—not always loud or commanding, but steady and confident. Roman-footed individuals often make great **mediators and decision-makers**, thanks to their even temperament and logical mindset.

3. Sociable & Friendly

They are often **outgoing, approachable, and charismatic**. Roman types enjoy **connection, conversation, and community**. While they value facts and fairness, they also like to be surrounded by people and are generally easy to get along with.

4. Balanced Thinkers

With the equal length of the top three toes, this foot shape represents **mental, emotional, and physical balance**. Roman types aim for equilibrium in life and are typically measured in their responses. They don't rush decisions and prefer a **structured approach** to challenges.

5. Loyal & Steady

Reliability is key—they are the ones others turn to for **support, logic, and follow-through**. They can carry burdens for others without complaint and are often **devoted friends, partners, and colleagues**.

6. Sensible but Curious

While they're grounded, Roman-footed individuals still have a **sense of curiosity and desire to explore**, especially in areas of culture, history, and systems. They're not easily swayed by fantasy but **thrive on meaningful experiences**.

Reflexology/Bodywork Tips for Roman Feet:

- **Pressure Preference:** Medium to firm pressure is usually welcomed; they enjoy structure and method.
- **Best Techniques:** Systematic thumb-walking, pressure-point release, and clear sequencing.
- **Connection Style:** Be professional and personable—they appreciate clarity, consistency, and a touch of warmth.
- **Healing Focus:** Encourage flexibility and emotional release—sometimes they carry more than they show and could benefit from Heart Chakra or Solar Plexus balancing.

Egyptian Foot Personality Tendencies

The **Egyptian foot shape**— characterized by a long, narrow foot with a **sloping toe line** (each toe shorter than the previous one, forming a gentle diagonal from the big toe to the smallest)—is the most commonly found shape in the population and carries unique energetic and personality traits.

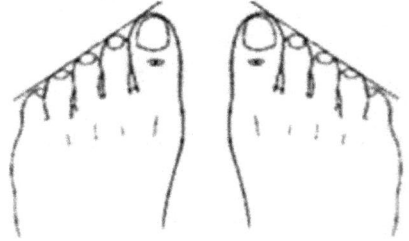

1. Dreamer & Visionary

People with Egyptian-shaped feet often have a **romantic, idealistic nature**. They are vision-driven individuals who prefer to look ahead to possibilities rather than dwell on limitations. This shape reflects someone who **thinks deeply** and **dreams big**.

2. Private & Reserved

The tapering shape suggests **privacy and discretion**. These individuals may be selective about who they open up to and tend to **keep their inner world hidden** unless trust is earned. They enjoy their personal space and time to process emotions.

3. Aesthetic Sensitivity

Often drawn to **beauty, design, and harmony**, Egyptian-footed clients may be **visually attuned** and appreciative of balance and elegance. They could be artists, stylists, or simply people who value ambiance and detail.

4. Gentle Energy

These individuals may not respond well to aggressive or abrupt approaches. They prefer **softer techniques** and benefit from **flowing, nurturing energy**—both physically in treatments and emotionally in conversations.

5. Idealists with High Standards

They may struggle when reality doesn't match their inner ideals. Egyptian-footed personalities often **expect a lot from themselves and others**, which can lead to **perfectionism** or occasional disappointment.

6. Spiritually Inclined

There is often a **spiritual or philosophical dimension** to their thinking. They seek deeper meaning in life and may be naturally drawn to **meditation, intuition, or metaphysical exploration**.

Reflexology/Bodywork Tips for Egyptian Feet:

- **Pressure Preference:** Gentle to medium pressure; avoid abrupt or overly firm movements at first.
- **Best Techniques:** Flowing strokes, circular thumb walking, and energy balancing work.
- **Connection Style:** Establish trust slowly—speak calmly, and allow space for quiet reflection.
- **Healing Focus:** Grounding techniques and Root Chakra support may be beneficial to offset their tendency to "float" into dreams or overthinking.

Germanic (Square) Foot Personality Tendencies

The **Germanic foot shape**, sometimes called the **Square Foot**, is defined by all **five toes being nearly the same length**, creating a boxy, broad appearance. It gives the foot a strong, grounded look and is less common than the Egyptian or Roman types.

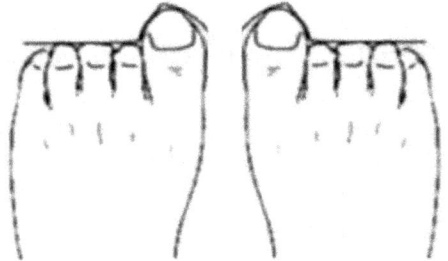

1. Logical & Analytical

People with Germanic-shaped feet tend to be **methodical thinkers**. They analyze situations carefully and prefer **facts over feelings** when making decisions. Their logic-based approach makes them excellent planners and problem solvers.

2. Grounded & Reliable

The balanced toe length reflects **stability, dependability, and a grounded presence**. These individuals tend to have **strong roots**, both in personality and in life. You can count on them to show up and follow through with what they say.

3. Practical & Realistic

They prefer **what works** over what looks good. This foot type belongs to someone who values **functionality, systems, and results**. They're often drawn to careers or lifestyles that require **efficiency, organization, and structure**.

4. Cautious & Reserved

Germanic-footed personalities usually **don't rush into things**. They like to observe, plan, and assess before taking action. While this can make them seem cautious or even stoic, it's actually a form of **internal strength and foresight**.

5. Honest & Straightforward

What you see is what you get. These individuals have a **no-nonsense communication style**—they prefer clear, honest dialogue and value **integrity and transparency** in others. They dislike manipulation or emotional games.

6. Emotionally Self-Contained

While not cold, they tend to be **more private with emotions**, often keeping their feelings to themselves unless they fully trust someone. Their energy is consistent and solid, not prone to highs and lows.

Reflexology/Bodywork Tips for Germanic Feet:

- **Pressure Preference:** Firm and steady—these feet are durable and respond well to structural work.
- **Best Techniques:** Consistent thumb walking, joint mobilization, and systematic reflex point engagement.
- **Connection Style:** Be clear and confident—these clients respect expertise and appreciate when sessions feel purposeful.
- **Healing Focus:** Help soften rigidity and increase flexibility—physically and emotionally. Liver and gallbladder meridians may need attention, as they tend to hold onto stress mentally rather than express it.

Celtic Foot Personality Tendencies

The **Celtic foot shape**—a lesser-known but energetically rich type—is characterized by a **long big toe, a shorter second toe, and then fluctuating lengths of the remaining toes**, often with the fourth toe dropping lower than the fifth. It can look a bit uneven or "irregular," which reflects its **uniquely complex energy signature**.

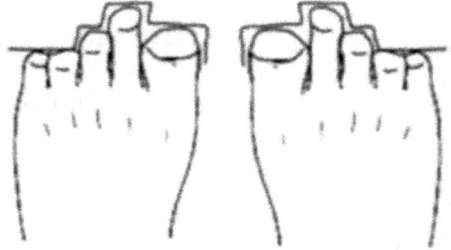

1. Intuitive & Deeply Feeling

Celtic-footed individuals are highly **emotionally attuned** and often deeply **intuitive**, even empathic. They feel the energy of others strongly and may need to **retreat** often to process all they absorb. Their foot shape reflects **emotional depth and psychic sensitivity**.

2. Creative & Expressive

There is an **artistic and poetic** streak in Celtic-footed people. They often see beauty in odd places and express their emotions through **writing, music, visual arts, or storytelling**. Their minds are imaginative, rich, and sometimes a little chaotic—but always meaningful.

3. Unique & Independent

This foot shape is rarely "symmetrical," which reflects a **free-spirited, nonconformist personality**. Celtic-footed clients don't do well being boxed in—they want the freedom to

explore, invent, and live authentically, even if it means going against the grain.

4. Sensitive to Stress

Their fluctuating toe length can symbolize **inner conflict or emotional fluctuations**. These individuals are **easily affected by stress**, especially from relationships, and may somaticize emotions into physical tension—especially in the neck, shoulders, and digestive system.

5. Loyal but Protective

They're **incredibly loyal** to the few they let into their inner world. However, Celtic personalities **guard their trust** fiercely. They may appear distant or skeptical at first, but once a connection is built, their care runs deep.

6. Old Soul Energy

There is often a sense of **ancient wisdom or "knowing"** about Celtic-footed individuals. They may have an interest in **ancestral lineage, folklore, mysticism, or the unseen realms**. Many are drawn to healing, spiritual work, or emotional counseling.

Reflexology/Bodywork Tips for Celtic Feet:

- **Pressure Preference:** Variable—check in frequently. One area may want soft nurturing touch, another firmer grounding work.
- **Best Techniques:** Energy flow balancing, reflex point holding (rather than constant motion), emotional release work, Reiki integration.
- **Connection Style:** Hold space for trust—these clients may need time before fully relaxing. Allow conversation or silence based on their lead.

- **Healing Focus:** Solar Plexus, Third Eye, and Sacral Chakra balancing. Work on integrating intuition with personal power, and grounding sensitive energy into the body.

2. Arch Height: Structural and Energetic Indicators

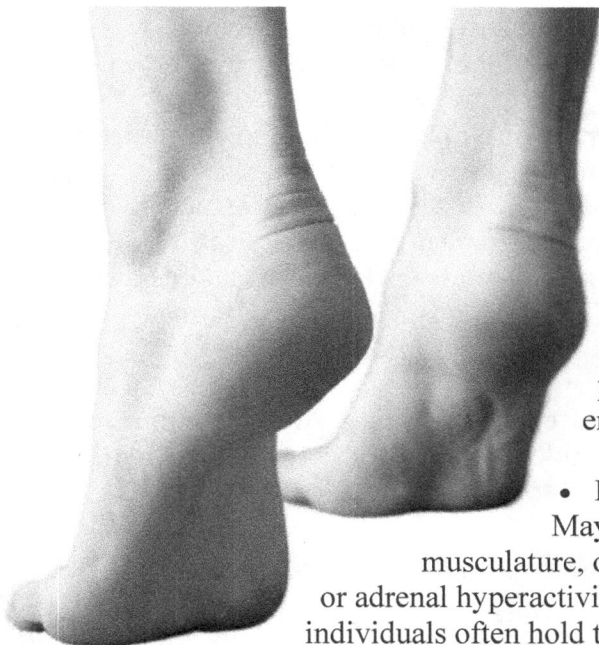

The arch of the foot plays a major role in weight distribution, shock absorption, and core stability. It also reflects internal tone—physically and emotionally.

- **High Arches** – May suggest tight musculature, overcompensation, or adrenal hyperactivity. These individuals often hold themselves in high alert and may benefit from grounding techniques.
- **Flat Feet** – Can indicate muscular fatigue, poor core engagement, or long-standing stress. Emotionally, it may suggest feeling unsupported or chronically burdened.
- **Collapsed Arches on One Side** – Often tied to unbalanced weight-bearing or chronic injury compensation. Can reflect emotional imbalance between giving and receiving.

Quick Check: Ask the client to stand barefoot. Look for weight distribution and pressure imprint from heel to toe.

3. Symmetry: Alignment & Functional Clues

Comparing both feet reveals a wealth of insight into compensation patterns and underlying asymmetries.

- **One foot larger or wider** – Often seen with structural imbalances in hips, knees, or scoliosis.
- **Different skin tone or texture** – May relate to circulation or lymphatic differences.
- **Muscle bulk or softness variation** – Suggests overuse or disuse of a particular side of the body, usually tied to dominant hand/leg or postural habits.

Observe posture seated and standing. Are the feet turned out equally? Does one ankle roll inward or outward? These offer clues about pelvic tilt, spinal curve, or knee stress.

4. Postural Clues: Footprints of Daily Life

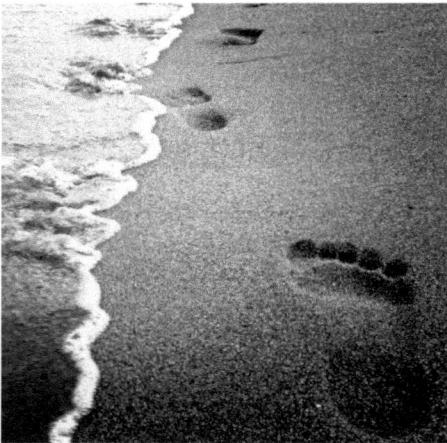

Feet act as the foundation for every step. Imbalances here ripple upward through the body, influencing gait, back pain, joint health, and even energy levels.

- **Toes that grip the floor** – Often associated with anxiety, hypervigilance, or the need for control.
- **Weight shifted toward heels** – Common in those who resist moving forward or who suppress emotion.
- **Pronated or supinated feet** – Reveal long-standing movement patterns that contribute to hip, shoulder, or jaw tension.

Advanced Insight: When feet point in opposite directions during rest or walking, it may suggest cross-body compensation or a history of physical/emotional trauma.

Putting It All Together

When you combine foot shape, arch height, symmetry, and postural signs, you gain a holistic picture of your client's body map. This isn't about labeling or diagnosing—but rather *witnessing* the story the feet tell and using that wisdom to guide your reflexology session with more attunement and impact.

Left vs. Right Foot: Emotional vs. Physical Perspective

In reflexology, the body is viewed as a dynamic interplay of energies—physical, emotional, mental, and spiritual. The **left and right feet**, while mirror images in anatomy, often represent *very different aspects* of a person's life and inner landscape.

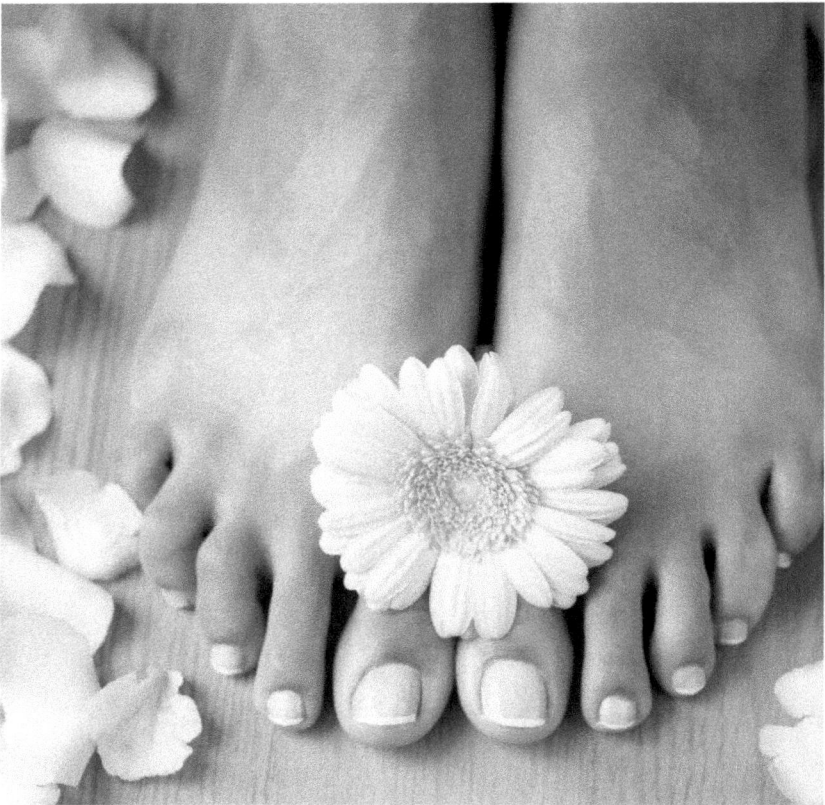

Understanding this polarity can help practitioners identify patterns that might otherwise go unnoticed and guide clients toward deeper self-awareness and healing.

The Left Foot: Emotional and Internal World

Traditionally, the **left side of the body**—and therefore the left foot—is associated with the **emotional, intuitive, and feminine** aspects of life. It governs:

- Inner processing and unresolved emotions
- Relationship with the self
- Maternal lineage and inherited emotional patterns
- Subconscious or unspoken issues
- Receptivity, creativity, and intuition

Clues from the Left Foot:

- Tenderness on the left side of a reflex zone may suggest an emotional root or suppressed feeling.
- Puffiness or excess heat on the left foot could indicate emotional inflammation, especially in zones like the heart, chest, or solar plexus.
- Repeated callusing or hollowness on the left may point to long-standing internal struggles or emotional shutdown.

The Right Foot: Physical and External World

The **right side of the body**—and thus the right foot—typically reflects the **action-oriented, logical, and masculine** side. It relates to:

- Physical health and tangible symptoms
- Responsibility, control, and structure
- Paternal lineage and societal expectations
- Decision-making and forward movement

- Expression and external relationships

Clues from the Right Foot:

- Sharp pain or congestion on the right foot often aligns with physical symptoms in the corresponding body area.
- Hardened areas may signal overexertion, stress from daily responsibilities, or long-term suppression of physical needs.
- A cooler temperature on the right may suggest energetic withdrawal or adrenal depletion.

Working with Both Feet Together

While each foot holds its own symbolic and practical information, **the relationship between both feet is key**. Asymmetry between them can reveal where a client may be disconnected—living in their head but ignoring their heart, or prioritizing others while neglecting their own emotional needs.

Example: A client may have sharp pain in the right kidney zone (physical stress overload) but a spongy, tender left kidney zone (emotional overwhelm). The combination points to both physical burnout and emotional depletion—likely from being in "survival mode" for too long.

Using This Insight in Sessions

As a practitioner:

- Start each session by noticing the balance between the two feet—do they feel energetically aligned?
- Ask neutral, open-ended questions if one side seems more reactive.
- Use this duality as a reflection tool: *"Do you feel like this situation is showing up more physically, emotionally, or both?"*

This left-right framework doesn't replace anatomical knowledge—it **enhances it**. When approached with curiosity, it becomes a doorway to whole-person healing and greater client self-awareness.

There is a strong symbolic and energetic **correlation between the left/right foot and the left/right hemispheres of the brain**, and it's deeply relevant in holistic and reflexology-based healing. Here's how it connects:

Brain Hemispheres and Foot Symbolism

Why the Brain Hemispheres Control the Opposite Side of the Body (Including the Feet)

This reversal is known as **contralateral control**, and it's a well-established principle in neuroanatomy.

Here's the short version:

- The **left hemisphere of the brain controls the right side** of the body.
- The **right hemisphere of the brain controls the left side** of the body.
- This applies to your **arms, legs, hands, and feet.**

The Scientific Reason

Inside the brainstem, there's a crossover point called the **decussation of the pyramids**, located in the **medulla oblongata** (part of the brainstem). At this point, the nerve fibers from the **motor cortex** (which controls movement) **cross over to the opposite side** before traveling down the spinal cord.

- So, motor commands from the **left brain** travel to the **right side of the body**, and vice versa.

- Sensory signals also typically **cross over**, meaning touch from the right foot is processed in the left hemisphere.

While the **left brain controls the right side of the body**, and the **right brain controls the left side**, the **traits of each hemisphere** also reflect the types of energy associated with each foot in reflexology.

Brain Hemisphere	Foot Connection	Associated Traits
Left Brain (Logical)	**Right Foot**	Rational thought, structure, order, speech, detail-focused, goal-oriented, control, masculine energy
Right Brain (Creative)	**Left Foot**	Emotions, intuition, creativity, imagination, big-picture thinking, empathy, feminine energy

Putting It Together in Reflexology Terms

- When the **right foot** shows stress (hardness, coldness, or congestion), the client may be **overextended in logical, outward, or responsibility-heavy aspects** of life—working too much, suppressing emotions, or pushing themselves to "perform."
- When the **left foot** shows imbalances (tender zones, puffiness, or holding patterns), it may suggest **emotional suppression, creative blocks, or unresolved internal conflict**—things that haven't been given conscious attention.

Reflexology and Energetic Healing Implications

In reflexology, this scientific reversal **symbolically aligns** with how we view **masculine/feminine** or **doing/feeling** energies:

Brain Hemisphere	Controls	Foot	Symbolic/Energetic Traits
Left	Right side of body	Right foot	Masculine, logical, structured, outer world
Right	Left side of body	Left foot	Feminine, emotional, creative, inner world

Case Application Example

A client has a stiff, hardened area on the **right foot's shoulder reflex**, with no visible physical injury. They report neck/shoulder tension from their office job. However, their **left shoulder reflex** feels spongy and warm—suggesting the emotional burden of holding in unexpressed frustrations.

You might say: *"It feels like you're physically carrying a lot on your shoulders, but there's something deeper here—do you often feel pressure to keep everything together, even emotionally?"*

As a Practitioner

Understanding the brain/foot connection helps you:

- **Balance left/right interpretations**—not all right foot issues are just physical; some are connected to left-brain overload.
- **Explore both hemispheres in sessions**: Ask questions that help clients reflect on both their **outer actions** (right brain/right foot) and **inner world** (left brain/left foot).
- **Support integration**: Reflexology naturally supports the communication between hemispheres, which enhances body-mind balance.

Why This Matters in Practice

When you feel something unusual on a client's **left foot**, it may suggest:

- Right hemisphere/emotional/creative imbalance
- Inner world, intuitive, or past emotional stress

When you feel something on the **right foot**, it may relate to:

- Left hemisphere/logical stress
- Outer world, action-based pressures, or over-control

The **cross-over between brain and body** isn't just a neurological fact—it's a map that reflexologists and energy healers can use to:

- Understand **deeper energetic imbalances**
- Ask more meaningful client questions
- Support **whole-body integration** (left + right, masculine + feminine, thinking + feeling)

Energetic Feel of the Feet

What Density, Warmth, and Responsiveness Reveal

Before words are spoken or reflex points are engaged, the **energetic feel** of a client's feet can offer a wealth of insight. As reflexologists and intuitive practitioners, we often "read" energy through our hands—long before logic gets involved.

Tuning into the **density, warmth, and responsiveness** of the feet is a foundational yet often overlooked skill in advanced reflexology.

Warmth vs. Coolness

- **Warm feet** often indicate healthy blood flow, grounded energy, and emotional openness.
- **Cool or cold feet** may suggest poor circulation, adrenal fatigue, energetic withdrawal, or even fear-based patterns (especially when the temperature difference is stark between feet).
- **One cold foot, one warm foot** may point to an imbalance between masculine and feminine energy, or between action and emotion.

Density and Tissue Quality

- **Heavy or dense-feeling feet** can suggest energetic stagnation, lymphatic congestion, or emotional heaviness.
- **Puffy or water-logged texture** often corresponds to poor elimination or unresolved emotional processing.

- **Light or soft feet** may reflect vitality, but in some cases may feel "ungrounded"—especially if paired with fidgety leg movement or tension in the hips.
- **Hard or rigid areas** might point to deep-seated holding patterns, often stored from trauma or long-standing stress.

Responsiveness to Touch

- **Highly reactive feet** (flinching, twitching, or sudden movement) might indicate heightened nervous system sensitivity, anxiety, or even trauma stored in specific reflex areas.
- **Feet that feel "numb" or energetically flat** can point to emotional dissociation, physical exhaustion, or suppressed expression.
- A **sinking-in feeling** under your hands may signal trust and release, whereas **resistance or tight recoil** may indicate guardedness—either physical or emotional.

Tip for Practitioners:

Pay attention not just to **what you feel under the skin**, but **what you feel through your hands**. Sometimes it's not a texture, but a presence—a message beneath the surface. Trust that your tactile sensitivity is a bridge between your client's body and their deeper energetic state.

This subtle awareness often tells the **real story** before the session has even begun.

Signs of Trauma, Exhaustion, or Disconnection

The feet often whisper what the client cannot yet say. Long before someone recognizes their own burnout, emotional shutdown, or past trauma, the body will attempt to reveal the truth—especially through the feet. These signs aren't just physical—they are **energetic footprints** of a story the nervous system still holds.

1. Trauma Imprints

Trauma leaves more than emotional scars—it creates **cellular memory**. The body stores these memories in muscles, fascia, and reflex zones.

Common indicators in the feet:

- **Hardened tissue** or **"armor-like" bands** around the ankles or top of foot
- **Flinching or recoil** during light pressure—especially over the spine, pelvic, or heart zones
- A **sharp, localized tenderness** that surprises the client or brings up unexpected emotion
- **One foot colder or more rigid** than the other (particularly the left side in emotional trauma)

Energetic note: These feet often "guard" themselves, even when the client presents as open. You may feel a barrier—like your hands can't connect deeply.

2. Exhaustion and Burnout

Clients who are energetically depleted may present with feet that feel:

- **Flat and unresponsive**, lacking the "bounce" of healthy tissue
- **Cold, clammy, or pallid**
- **Dry and cracked**, especially around heels and balls of feet (linked to adrenal fatigue and overextension)
- **Sinking quickly into your touch** as if the body is silently begging for help

Clients may report symptoms like:

- "I'm always tired, even after sleep."
- "I feel like I'm running on fumes."
- "Nothing seems to recharge me anymore."

3. Disconnection or Dissociation

When someone is not fully "in their body," the feet often show it.

Telltale signs include:

- A **rubbery**, almost **lifeless feel** to the foot (despite normal blood flow)
- **Lack of temperature change** during the session, even when circulation should be stimulated
- Feet feel **heavy but energetically absent**—like your hands are touching something without "presence"
- The client avoids eye contact or seems mentally "checked out" during the session

These feet don't just need pressure—they need permission to come back into the body gently.

Practitioner Insight

When working with clients showing these signs:

- **Slow down** your session pace
- Use **softer transitions** and grounding holds
- Encourage **breathwork** and quiet presence
- Never push emotional release—allow the body to lead

You don't need to label trauma, diagnose burnout, or define the story. The role of the reflexologist is to **witness, support, and create space**—so that healing can occur in its own time.

Let the feet tell you what the client may not be ready to say.

Chapter 4: Toe Talk – What the Toes Reveal

Toes are tiny storytellers.

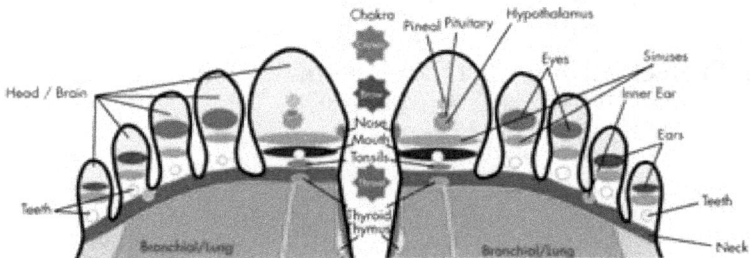

They may seem like the smallest detail in a reflexology session, but toes offer profound insights into how a person processes stress, carries tension, and expresses themselves— emotionally, mentally, and even spiritually.

When you pay attention to the shape, movement, and surface of the toes, you're reading into years of postural adaptation, trauma, habit, and energetic imprinting.

Calluses on Toes

Calluses are more than friction from footwear. They're the body's way of armoring itself. When found on the toes, they often relate to **overuse, guarding, or emotional suppression** tied to the reflex zones of the affected toes.

- **Big Toe Callus (Brain & Head Zone):** Mental overdrive, worry loops, decision fatigue. Often seen in perfectionists or overthinkers.
- **Second Toe (Eyes & Sinuses):** Strained vision (literal or metaphorical), often found in people struggling to "see" their next steps.
- **Third Toe (Ears, Neck):** Communication blocks or listening fatigue. Clients may say, "I'm tired of everyone's noise."
- **Fourth Toe (Shoulder, Upper Back):** Emotional burden or pressure to "carry others." Common in caregivers or those with upper back pain.
- **Fifth Toe (Pelvis, Lymphatic):** Repressed sexuality or creative energy. Often callused and tucked under in clients who have experienced shame or body discomfort.

Curvature and Toe Positioning

The alignment of the toes reveals how energy flows through the body—and where it gets stuck.

- **Hammer Toes:** Suggest long-held tension, often linked to anxiety or self-protection. These clients "grip" life with their toes, rarely feeling grounded.
- **Claw Toes or Contractures:** Chronic over-efforting. The client may feel like they must always be "on guard." Often accompanied by adrenal burnout.
- **Crossed Toes:** Emotional entanglement or unresolved tension with others. When toes twist over each other, look for stories of caretaking, codependency, or relational overwhelm.
- **Toes Spread Wide Apart:** Independence, strong-willed personality, open communication style. Often seen in clients who "walk their own path."
- **Toes Squeezed Close Together**: Need for control, protection, or hiding. These feet often come with

comments like "I hate my feet" or visible self-consciousness.

Toe Spacing and Emotional Themes

Each toe represents different energetic expressions:

Toe	Reflex Connection	Energetic Insight
Big Toe	Brain, Pineal, Pituitary	Mental activity, decision-making
Second Toe	Eyes, Sinuses	Vision, perception
Third Toe	Ears, Neck	Communication, receptivity
Fourth Toe	Shoulder	Emotional responsibility
Fifth Toe	Pelvic, Reproductive	Security, creativity

If one toe is significantly shorter, curled, or tucked under, it can symbolize **a blocked area in that expression**.

What Toe Pain May Reveal

Pain isn't random. In the toes, it often reflects both **current physical stress** and **suppressed or unresolved emotional tension**. Each toe is associated with a particular reflex zone and energetic archetype, so pain or tenderness can act as an internal alarm bell.

Big Toe (Head, Brain, Pineal/Pituitary Glands)

Common Pain Patterns: Throbbing, tension, nerve sensitivity

- **Physical Indications:** Headaches, migraines, hormonal imbalances, sleep issues
- **Emotional Correlates:** Overthinking, decision fatigue, mental burnout, lack of clarity
- **Client Expressions:** "I feel mentally foggy," "I can't stop thinking about it."

Second Toe (Eyes, Sinuses, Neck)

- **Common Pain Patterns:** Sharp pain or numbness
- **Physical Indications:** Visual stress, sinus pressure, eye strain
- **Emotional Correlates:** Inability to see one's path clearly, internal conflict
- **Client Expressions:** "I feel stuck and can't see the way forward."

Third Toe (Ears, Throat, Neck)

- **Common Pain Patterns:** Burning sensation or tension
- **Physical Indications:** TMJ, stiff neck, communication challenges
- **Emotional Correlates:** Fear of speaking up, feeling unheard, inner conflict
- **Client Expressions:** "I keep biting my tongue," "No one listens to me."

Fourth Toe (Shoulder, Upper Back)

- **Common Pain Patterns:** Dull aching, sensitivity to pressure
- **Physical Indications:** Shoulder tension, frozen shoulder, back strain
- **Emotional Correlates:** Carrying burdens, emotional weight, guilt or obligation
- **Client Expressions:** "It feels like I carry the world on my shoulders."

Fifth Toe (Reproductive, Pelvis, Lymphatics)

- **Common Pain Patterns:** Numbness, cramping, stiffness
- **Physical Indications:** Hip pain, pelvic floor tension, lymphatic stagnation
- **Emotional Correlates:** Suppressed creativity, safety fears, body image issues, sexual repression
- **Client Expressions:** "I feel disconnected from my lower body," "I've shut that part of myself off."

Pain as a Message, Not a Diagnosis

While pain in the toes shouldn't be used to diagnose a condition, it can:

- **Alert you** to areas needing deeper attention.
- **Reveal stored trauma** or repetitive stress.
- **Guide session flow**—often the most tender toes point to the area where healing wants to begin.

How to Work with Toe Pain in Sessions

- Use **gentle alternating pressure**—never force.
- Ask: "Do you recognize any recent stress or strain in this part of your body or life?"
- Avoid labeling—stay curious.
- After working the toes, recheck sensitivity. Often, pain decreases mid-session if you're accessing the right reflexes.

Practitioner Tip:

Use the toes as conversation openers. Not with assumptions, but with gentle invitations:

"Your toes are showing me a lot today—do you ever feel like your body holds tension before your mind catches on?"

Optional Support Suggestions:

- **Soak and release tension** with Epsom salt or magnesium foot baths.
- **Stretch and spread toes** daily to increase circulation and release held energy.
- Recommend **yoga for feet**, grounding walks, or wearing toe spacers if alignment is tight or painful.

Hammer Toes, Morton's Toe, and Overlapping Toes

Structural signs that speak volumes about postural habits, emotional holding patterns, and deeper systemic imbalances.

Morton's Toe

What it looks like: The second toe is longer than the big toe. Common in 20–30% of the population.

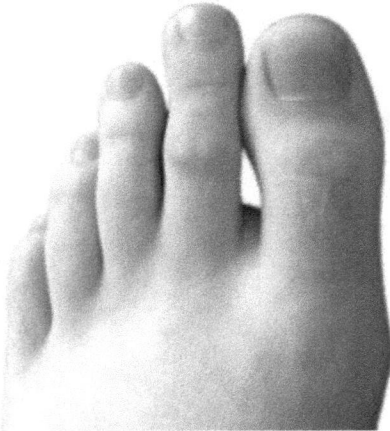

Reflexology meaning:

- **Biomechanical Compensation:** This affects gait and posture, often leading to knee, hip, or back issues over time.

- **Leadership/Responsibility Archetype:** Often seen in clients who carry a lot of responsibility or take on leadership roles (whether by choice or necessity).
- **Energetic Imbalance:** This toe may absorb stress from multiple reflex zones (spine, neck, eyes, sinus)— especially if callused or inflamed.

Common client confirmations:

- Shoulder pain, hip imbalance, plantar fasciitis.
- Stress-related disorders due to high expectations or personal pressure.
- "I always have to be the one to step up."

Hammer Toes

What it looks like: One or more toes bend downward at the middle joint, often becoming rigid or unable to lie flat on the ground.

Reflexology meaning:

- **Cervical Spine Stress:** Hammer toes often correlate with neck and upper spine tension, especially when affecting the 2nd and 3rd toes.
- **Chronic Mental Tension:** Clients may be overthinkers or carry persistent worry in their mental field.
- **Energetic Holding:** This toe shape often suggests rigidity—mentally, emotionally, or energetically. It may reflect someone who is "always bracing for something."

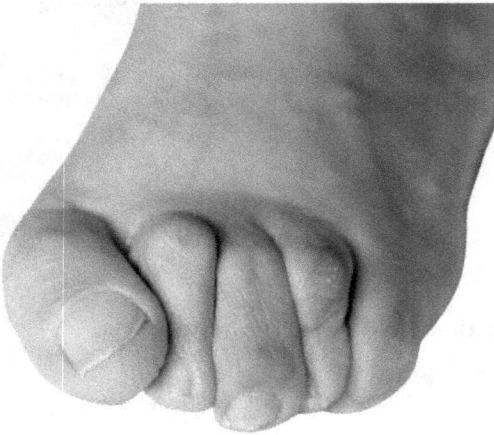

Common client confirmations:

- Tension headaches, migraines, neck pain.
- Personality traits of perfectionism or needing to control outcomes.

- Long hours at a desk, driving, or looking down at devices.

Overlapping Toes

What it looks like: One toe crosses or rests on top of another, commonly the 2nd or 4th over the 3rd.

Reflexology meaning:

- **Emotional Conflict or Suppression:** Overlapping toes often symbolize inner conflict or a part of the self being "silenced" or overridden by another.
- **Trauma or Developmental Pattern:** May develop in early childhood due to womb position, tight footwear, or inherited structure.
- **Energetic Imprint:** Suggests repression, layered emotional experiences, or lack of personal space.

Common client confirmations:

- Family tension, people-pleasing, unexpressed emotions.
- History of "shrinking to fit in" or being overpowered by others.
- May also correlate with TMJ tension, pelvic misalignment, or difficulty expressing needs.

Supportive Actions

Bodywork & Movement:

- **Chiropractic or craniosacral therapy** to address structural misalignment.
- **Reflexology & massage** to soften compensatory tension.
- **Yoga or Pilates** to improve posture, breath, and gait.

Emotional Healing:

- Explore journaling questions like:
  - ○ "Where do I feel pressured to conform?"
  - ○ "What part of myself feels hidden or overridden?"
- Energy healing or somatic therapy to release held emotional patterns.

Foot Care & Shoes:

- Encourage barefoot walking on natural surfaces (when safe).
- Switch to wide toe-box, zero-drop shoes to prevent further compression.

Dental Links: Dorsal Toe Bumps and Orthodontic Trauma

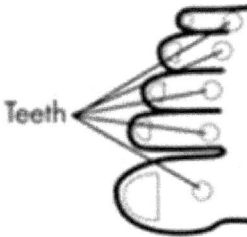

*H*ow *the feet may reveal the energetic residue of dental procedures—especially along the dorsal (top) surfaces of the toes.*

What to Look For

- **Hard bumps or small calluses** on the **top (dorsal) side** of the toes—especially the second, third, and fourth toes.
- May be **centered over joints** or appear as ridges between toe knuckles.
- Texture may feel **dense, gritty, or sharp-edged** to the reflexologist's thumb.

Possible Reflexology Meanings

These dorsal toe bumps frequently correspond to:

- **Dental trauma or residual tension** from:
  - Braces and retainers
  - Tooth extractions or root canals
  - Crowns, implants, or jaw surgery
  - TMJ dysfunction
- **Energetic blocks** from disrupted facial meridians or cranial reflex points.

The top of the toes—especially the middle three—correlate reflexively to:

- **Sinuses** (front of toe)
- **Teeth, jaw, and facial nerves** (central toe joints)
- **Brain and cranial reflexes** (base of toes and under nail beds)

Energetic and Emotional Insight

Dental procedures often involve:

- **Long periods of holding tension** in the jaw
- **Suppression of expression** (especially during orthodontic work in youth)
- **Energetic fragmentation** (due to invasive interventions in the head/face region)

These dorsal toe signs can represent:

- **Unresolved trauma** stored in the craniofacial nervous system
- **Energetic short-circuiting** between communication centers (throat chakra) and emotional control centers (jaw, solar plexus)
- **A need to "bite down" emotionally**—showing restraint, silence, or control

Common Client Confirmations

Clients with dorsal toe bumps often say things like:

- "I had braces for years as a teen."
- "I clench my jaw at night and didn't realize it."
- "I've had multiple root canals on the same side."
- "I had dental trauma as a child and still hate going to the dentist."

- "I get tension headaches or earaches that start in my jaw."

Complementary Support Suggestions

Body & Structural Support:

- **Craniosacral therapy** or **TMJ massage** to release stored jaw and facial tension
- **Dental referral** if pain, bite imbalance, or gum issues are reported
- **Chiropractic care** if postural patterns stem from jaw-to-neck misalignment

Energetic Healing:

- Reiki or sound healing focused on the **throat and jaw chakras**
- Guided imagery or meditation for **voice reclamation**
- Acupressure points for jaw release (e.g., SI19, ST6, GB2)

Emotional Work:

- Journaling prompts like:
  - "Where have I had to stay silent to stay safe?"
  - "What truths do I still need to speak?"
- Emotional release techniques for early childhood experiences tied to braces or dental pain

Neurological or Emotional Tension in Curled or Rigid Toes

What chronically tense, curled, or rigid toes reveal about the nervous system and emotional holding patterns.

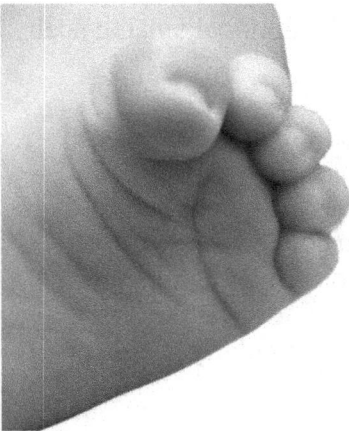

What to Look For

- **Toes that curl downward or under**, even at rest
- Toes that feel **stiff or inflexible** when manipulated
- **Rigid toe joints** that resist movement or feel locked
- **Overlapping toes**, often combined with tightness or deformity
- Toes that **lift off the ground** unnaturally (indicative of muscular imbalance or instability)

Reflexology and Structural Meaning

Each toe represents both **a physical zone** and **an emotional or neurological reflection** of the client's inner world.

- **Big toe**: Head, brain, and decision-making
- **2nd toe**: Neck, eyes, personal direction
- **3rd toe**: Shoulders, elbows, self-carrying
- **4th toe**: Hips, knees, flexibility in action
- **5th toe**: Ears, communication, survival instincts

Curled or rigid toes may indicate:

- **Cervical spine tension** or neurological compression
- **Peripheral nerve restriction**, particularly in diabetics or neuropathy clients
- **Postural imbalance** stemming from the hips, knees, or back
- **Overactive sympathetic nervous system** ("fight or flight" dominance)

Emotional or Energetic Meaning

These patterns often suggest long-held emotional tension such as:

- **Hypervigilance** – the nervous system is "on guard," creating rigidity in the body
- **Perfectionism or control issues** – especially if toes are held tightly in symmetrical tension
- **Fear of letting go** – toes curl or grip as a metaphor for emotional clenching
- **Suppressed grief or shame** – particularly if tension is asymmetrical or isolated to one foot

Energetically, curled toes can reflect:

- A lack of **grounding** or fear of vulnerability
- Unresolved trauma stored in **muscle memory**
- Patterns of **"standing alone" or feeling unsupported**

Common Client Confirmations

Clients with curled or rigid toes frequently confirm:

- A history of **stress, anxiety, PTSD**, or **over-responsibility**
- **Tension headaches, TMJ**, or **neck/shoulder pain**

- Emotional statements such as:
  - "I've always felt I had to be in control."
  - "I can't let my guard down."
  - "I carry everything on my shoulders."
  - "Even when I sleep, I'm tight."

Complementary Support Options

Neurological & Structural:

- **Reflexology** to stimulate relaxation and parasympathetic response
- **Chiropractic or osteopathic care** for spine and neck alignment
- **Stretching or yoga**, especially for toes, calves, and hamstrings
- **Neuromuscular massage** or **PNF stretching** to reset muscle memory

Emotional & Energetic Support:

- **Somatic therapy** to explore how emotions are stored in the body
- **Reiki** or **craniosacral therapy** to soothe hyperactive nerves
- **Grounding exercises** like barefoot walking, breathwork, or tapping
- Journaling prompts:
  - "Where in my life am I holding on too tightly?"
  - "What would happen if I allowed support?"

White Glow Beneath Toenails

(Brain Stress or Trauma)

*S*ubtle signs that may reveal neurological strain, past head injuries, or cognitive overload.

What It Looks Like

- A **pearly or milky-white glow** beneath the toenail, most often seen on the **big toes**
- Appears **not as surface discoloration** (like fungal issues) but as a **luminescent cast from underneath**
- Sometimes **only visible under strong light or after a foot soak**

Reflexology Meaning

In foot reflexology, the **big toes correspond to the brain, head, and upper neck**, including:

- The cerebral cortex
- Pituitary and pineal glands
- Hypothalamus
- Upper cervical spine and brain stem

When a **white glow** appears beneath the nail, it may indicate:

- **Neurological strain**, especially from overstimulation, chronic stress, or EMF sensitivity
- **History of head trauma**, such as concussions, whiplash, or birth trauma

- **Mental burnout** from overthinking, high-pressure decision-making, or unresolved emotional loops
- In some cases, it may reflect **inflammation in the brain** or cerebrospinal fluid imbalance (as reported anecdotally in TCM and energy work)

Energetic & Emotional Interpretation

Energetically, a white glow may represent:

- **Mental overload** or "white noise" in the mind
- **Overactivity of the crown or third eye chakra**, sometimes due to spiritual bypassing or intellectual overexertion
- A soul that's **"out of body" too often**, disconnected from grounding

Emotionally, this often correlates with:

- Clients who say, "I can't shut my brain off."
- People with histories of **perfectionism**, **sleeplessness**, or **anxiety loops**
- Individuals recovering from **emotional shock** or **mental trauma**

Client Confirmations

Clients with this sign have often shared:

- A history of **concussions, car accidents**, or **blows to the head**
- Intense **mental stress**, often in professions requiring high cognitive load (e.g., lawyers, engineers, healers)
- **Memory issues, brain fog**, or chronic **insomnia**
- In one case, a client with a longstanding white glow later disclosed a **benign brain tumor** diagnosed months after the reflexology session

Support Options

Physical & Neurological:

- **Craniosacral therapy** to regulate cerebrospinal fluid and calm the brain
- **Neurotherapy** or **biofeedback** for trauma resolution
- **Omega-3 supplementation**, B-vitamins, magnesium for cognitive support
- **Chiropractic care** for upper cervical spine

Energetic & Emotional:

- **Reiki to the head and crown**, with focus on grounding
- **Meditation practices** that quiet the mind (e.g., Yoga Nidra, sound baths)
- **Foot soaks with Himalayan salt or magnesium** to draw energy downward
- Journaling prompts:
    - "What mental weight am I carrying?"
    - "Where am I resisting rest?"
    - "What am I afraid will happen if I stop thinking?"

Chapter 5: The Ball of the Foot – Heart, Lungs, and Stress Holding

Redness, Puffiness, and Stress Patterns

The **ball of the foot** is a powerful reflex region associated with the **chest cavity**, particularly the **heart, lungs, thymus gland, and diaphragm**. It also reflects how a person holds stress—both **emotionally and physically**—in their upper body.

When assessing this area, practitioners often observe **three key indicators**: **redness**, **puffiness**, and distinct **tissue stress patterns**. These signs can appear long before a client discloses any related symptoms, making them an essential diagnostic layer in holistic reflexology.

Redness: Fire, Inflammation & Emotional Charge

What it looks like:
– Bright red or flushed areas
– Often warm to the touch
– May appear more prominently after long periods of standing or emotional stress

Possible meanings:
– **Heart strain** – especially from emotional heartbreak, overexertion, or blood pressure issues
– **Lung inflammation** – especially in smokers or clients with asthma or chronic bronchitis
– **Emotional overload** – anger, grief, or anxiety can all trigger energy heat in this zone
– **Thymus stimulation** – related to immune stress or immune system overdrive (autoimmunity)

Support Options:
– Heart-calming Reiki (heart chakra)
– Breathwork or vagus nerve activation
– Anti-inflammatory support (herbs: hawthorn, motherwort, adaptogens)
– Emotional release techniques (EFT, somatic journaling)

Puffiness: Congestion, Grief & Suppression

What it looks like:
– Spongy or thickened tissue
– Loss of definition in ball-of-foot contour
– Often cool to the touch, or alternates between cold and hot

Possible meanings:
– **Lymphatic stagnation in the chest cavity**
– **Unprocessed grief**, especially tied to loss, betrayal, or long-term sadness
– **Suppressed breath** – shallow breathing, anxiety, or trauma held in the diaphragm
– **Allergic reactions or sinus overload** may also reflect here if the upper lungs are inflamed

Support Options:
– Manual lymph drainage (or reflex lymph techniques)
– Grief support therapy, breath therapy, or emotional bodywork
– Deep diaphragmatic breathing (with guidance if trauma-based)
– Herbal teas: mullein, marshmallow root, lungwort, linden

Stress Patterns: Hardened Zones, Cracks, or Sensitivity

What it feels like under the hands:
– Dense, tight fascia under the pads of the feet
– Gritty or ropey texture
– Sharp tenderness in the center of the ball (especially right foot = heart reflex)

What it may indicate:
– **Chronic tension in the chest muscles or upper spine**
– **Postural stress** from hunching (desk work, caregiving, grief posture)
– **Emotional armoring** – a protective hardening to prevent vulnerability
– **Circulatory sluggishness** or shallow breath habits

Signs to correlate:
– Tight shoulders, jaw clenching, or upper back pain
– Recent emotional upheaval, especially involving relationships or family
– History of bronchitis, pneumonia, or heart palpitations

Energetic Insights

The **ball of the foot** is like an emotional shield. When it's soft and responsive, the client is usually emotionally present and breathing deeply. But when it's dense, inflamed, or puffed, it's often storing years of stress, sadness, or self-protection.

On an energetic level:
– **Left foot** = emotional heart (loss, vulnerability, sadness)
– **Right foot** = physical heart (overload, pressure, responsibility)

Client Confirmations

Many clients have validated these observations:

- "That spot is always sore—it's where I clench when I'm stressed."
- "I've had heart palpitations lately…how did you know?"
- "I never realized how much I hold my breath until now."
- "I've been grieving my mother's death for years. It's all there."

Vertical Callus Between Toes

Acid Reflux & Digestive Stress

A vertical callus or **thickened ridge of skin** between the **1st and 2nd toes**—especially at the upper webbing or slightly beneath—can be a subtle but consistent **indicator of digestive imbalance**, most notably **acid reflux** or **upper GI stress**.

What It Looks/Feels Like:

- A **narrow, raised callus** that runs vertically rather than across the skin
- Often appears **slightly discolored** (yellowish or gray tone)
- May be **dry or tough** to the touch, but not painful unless irritated
- Can be **one-sided** (often right foot) or **bilateral**

Energetic & Reflex Meaning:

- This area corresponds to the **esophagus and upper stomach reflex zones** in reflexology.
- According to **Traditional Chinese Medicine (TCM)**, this part of the foot is linked to the **Stomach and Spleen meridians**, which govern digestion and assimilation.
- The skin's attempt to **"harden" or "buffer"** this area may reflect the body's chronic reaction to internal irritation—especially the upward movement of acidic digestive fluids.

What It May Indicate:

- **Chronic acid reflux (GERD)**
- **Hiatal hernia tension**
- **Burping, bloating, or indigestion**
- **Stress-related eating or emotional digestion issues**
- **Suppression of voice or swallowing emotions** (in psychosomatic terms)

Support Options:

- **Reflexology focus** on the diaphragm, solar plexus, stomach, and esophagus zones
- **Nutritional support**: alkaline foods, smaller meals, digestive bitters (with practitioner guidance)
- **Postural correction**: Elevating the head during sleep, avoiding slouching after meals
- **Stress relief practices**: especially vagus nerve activation and mindful eating
- **Herbal remedies**: chamomile, slippery elm, marshmallow root for gut lining support

Practitioner Notes:

- Check if the client has **a history of reflux, indigestion, or tight chest breathing**.
- If this area is **sensitive upon touch**, go gently and integrate diaphragm release through the solar plexus zone.
- If paired with **redness on the ball of the foot**, it may suggest **emotional tension** contributing to digestive symptoms.

Lung Area Signs

Asthma, Bronchitis, Smoking History

The **lung reflex zones** are primarily located on the **ball of the foot**, especially beneath the **pads of the toes** on both feet, slightly more centralized and medial (toward the inside). These zones are some of the most **communicative** when it comes to respiratory health—both past and present.

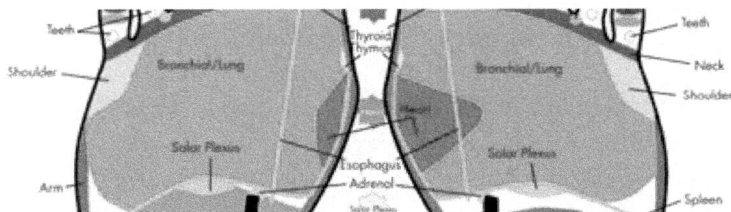

What to Look For in the Lung Reflex Zones:

1. Puffiness or Swelling

- **Spongy or thickened texture** in the ball of the foot.
- May indicate **congestion**—especially mucus buildup or chronic inflammation.
- Common in individuals with **asthma, bronchitis**, or **recurrent chest infections**.

2. Gritty or Sandy Texture

- Feels like **tiny pebbles or sugar grains** beneath the skin.
- Often linked to **old phlegm, poor lymphatic drainage**, or **toxic accumulation** from smoking.
- Indicates stagnation or incomplete clearing of the lungs after illness.

3. Hardened Calluses or Thick Skin

- Found particularly under the **4th and 5th toes**, outer ball of the foot.
- Frequently seen in **former smokers** or those exposed to secondhand smoke.
- Also common in clients with **COPD, emphysema**, or chronic environmental exposure (e.g., construction, pollution).

4. Redness or Warmth

- Active **inflammatory responses**, often acute.
- Seen during **allergy season, respiratory infections**, or emotional stress (lungs correlate with grief in TCM).
- May be accompanied by **shortness of breath** or upper chest tightness.

5. Hollowed Zones

- Especially near the **upper arch** where the lung zones blend with the diaphragm area.
- Can reflect **collapsed alveoli** (as in post-COVID or long-term bronchitis) or **energetic depletion** in breath capacity.
- May be seen in individuals who have suffered **grief**, deep sorrow, or chronic sadness.

Related Conditions These Signs May Reflect:

- Asthma (esp. if zones feel tight, inflamed, or tender)
- Bronchitis (puffy + gritty texture)
- Long COVID / post-viral lung recovery
- Smoking history (callused, gritty, hardened zones)
- Allergies (temporary puffiness + redness)
- Grief or breath-holding patterns (hollow or energetically dull zones)

Supportive Reflexology Approaches:

- **Diaphragm sweep** to open breathing
- Work the **lung, bronchial, sinus, and lymph** zones in sequence
- Include **solar plexus** and **adrenal reflexes** to reduce stress-related breath constriction

Complementary Therapies:

- **Breathwork** (especially vagus nerve-stimulating or nasal breathing techniques)
- **Lung-supportive herbs**: mullein, lobelia, elecampane
- **Lymphatic massage or dry brushing**
- **Hydration therapy** to thin mucus
- **Emotional processing** of grief (journaling, energy work, heart-lung integration meditations)

Practitioner Insight:

If the client is a **former smoker**, ask whether they've had a chest X-ray or lung capacity test if symptoms persist. Many people are unaware of **residual inflammation** even years after quitting. Reflexology can be deeply supportive in **clearing stagnant energy** and restoring breath vitality.

Heart Lines and Emotional Weight

In reflexology, the **heart reflex zone** is located on the **left foot**, specifically on the **ball of the foot just below the big toe and toward the medial (inner) side**. The **right foot** does not have a traditional heart reflex, though emotional indicators may still appear. What many reflexologists and energy-sensitive practitioners observe are **"heart lines"**—fine or deep **creases, cracks, or ridges**—appearing in or near this zone. These lines often reveal **emotional burdens, heart strain**, or unprocessed grief.

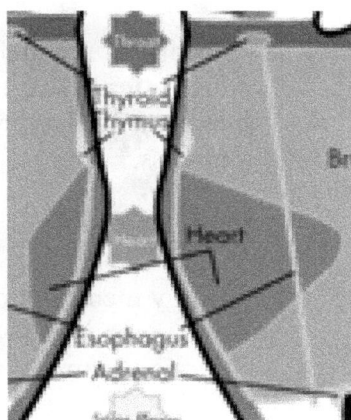

What Are Heart Lines?

Heart lines are:

- **Indented markings**, usually horizontal or diagonal.
- Sometimes **single and deep**, other times **multiple and faint**.
- Most visible in the **left foot** but can cross into both feet if emotional trauma is extensive.

They may appear:

- Just **beneath the ball** of the foot.
- **Under the big toe**, blending into thyroid or brain reflex zones.

- On the **medial arch**, trailing downward if emotional weight is long-held or internalized.

What They May Indicate

1. Emotional Stress or Grief

- The heart is intimately linked with **grief, heartbreak, and emotional suppression**.
- Lines may form after **loss, divorce**, or **prolonged loneliness**.

2. Heart Chakra Imbalance

- In energy medicine, deep lines here can suggest **closed-heartedness, difficulty giving/receiving love**, or **self-protection from vulnerability**.

3. Cardiovascular Strain

- While reflexology isn't diagnostic, deep markings in the heart zone may correlate with:
  - **High blood pressure**
  - **Poor circulation**
  - **Past cardiovascular events**
- Clients sometimes report a history of **angina, palpitations**, or **chest tightness** when these lines are noted.

4. Generational Heartache

- In some cases, the line doesn't feel "personal" to the client—they may carry **inherited emotional burdens** from parents or grandparents (a concept supported by ancestral healing or epigenetics).

Texture Clues Around Heart Lines:

- **Gritty texture** = energetic or lymphatic stagnation in the chest
- **Puffiness around the line** = emotional weight still held; unresolved grief
- **Callus overlaying the line** = guarded heart; long-term emotional self-protection
- **Hollowed area near the line** = depletion or emotional fatigue

How Practitioners Can Respond:

- **Gentle circular pressure** on the heart zone, supported by deep breathing prompts
- Include the **diaphragm reflex** to open emotional and physical breath
- Engage **Reiki or energetic intention** around the heart chakra (especially on the left side)
- Offer space to **talk or reflect**—clients often begin opening up emotionally after this zone is activated

Suggestions for Clients:

- Journaling prompt: *"What am I still holding in my heart?"*
- Encourage **forgiveness practices**, **breathwork**, or **heart-centered meditation**
- Emotional support remedies: **rose quartz, flower essences** (like Bleeding Heart or Willow), or **heart-opening teas** (e.g., hawthorn, rose)

Clinical Example:

A client with deep, horizontal lines across the heart reflex area once shared she'd never fully grieved her husband's passing five years earlier. After several sessions, the lines became less defined, and she reported improved sleep and a lighter chest feeling.

These markings are powerful emotional messengers. By gently working the **heart lines**, we support clients in **unburdening the emotional body**—sometimes without them even needing to speak.

Chapter 6: The Arch – Digestion, Liver, and Energy Reserves

Gritty Texture

Colon/Kidney Overload

In reflexology, the **arch of the foot**—stretching from the ball to the heel—mirrors the **core digestive and elimination organs**, including the **stomach, pancreas, liver, kidneys, small and large intestines, and adrenal glands**. When this area feels **gritty or sandy** to the touch, it often signals **toxic buildup, congestion**, or **stress in the body's detoxification systems**—particularly the **colon and kidneys**.

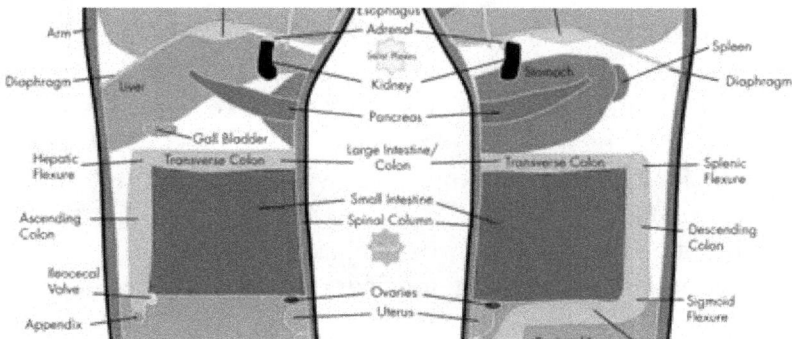

What the Gritty Texture Feels Like

To the practitioner, it may feel like:

- Fine **sand under the skin**
- Small **crystalline bumps**
- Subtle **crunchy resistance** when gliding over tissue
- Audible **grit-like sound** during movement

Clients may feel:

- Mild tenderness or discomfort
- A sense of "something releasing" as it's worked
- A surprising **urge to eliminate (bowel or urinary)** after the session

What It May Indicate:

Colon Overload

- Sluggish or incomplete elimination
- Chronic or subclinical **constipation, IBS**, or **bloating**
- Overconsumption of processed foods or low-fiber diets
- Emotional "holding" in the gut, often linked with **fear or control**

Kidney Stress

- Dehydration or excessive stimulant intake (e.g., caffeine, sugar)
- Difficulty filtering toxins (seen with fatigue, skin issues, or edema)
- Emotional links to **fear** (root chakra imbalance)
- Chronic low back pain or urinary discomfort

Liver Congestion

- Not as directly gritty, but may accompany texture changes in the arch
- Detox burden, especially with medications, alcohol, or emotional repression (anger)
- May present as **heaviness, thickened skin**, or **tenderness** in the medial arch

Common Causes of Gritty Texture

- Poor hydration
- High toxic load (environmental, dietary, emotional)
- Sedentary lifestyle (affecting lymphatic flow)
- Stress-related shutdown of digestive function
- Long-term suppression of emotions (especially anger, fear, or anxiety)

How to Work This Area

- Use **thumb-walking or circular gliding** techniques over gritty zones
- Encourage deep breathing during pressure for release
- Follow with work on the **kidney and bladder reflexes** to promote drainage
- Support with **Reiki**, especially over sacral and root chakra zones for elimination

Client Aftercare Suggestions

- **Hydration** with electrolyte-rich water post-session
- **Herbal teas** (dandelion, nettle, parsley) for kidney and colon cleansing
- **Gentle movement** like walking, yoga twists, or rebounding to stimulate lymph
- **Epsom salt foot soak** or full detox bath to draw out impurities

- Journaling prompt: *"What am I ready to let go of—physically or emotionally?"*

Emotional Symbolism

In energetic healing, the **arch holds the body's emotional "middle ground."** A gritty texture here may point to:

- Feeling **weighed down** by unprocessed experiences
- **Emotional stagnation** held in the gut (especially from grief, fear, or shame)
- Suppressed creativity or **burnout**—particularly if paired with low adrenal zones

Clinical Insight

In multiple clients with gritty arch texture:

- Those with **constipation** or sluggish bowels reported improvement after targeted footwork
- Clients with **frequent UTIs or kidney stones** often had gritty areas at the medial arch
- Highly stressed clients, especially those under pressure to "hold it together," often presented with both grit and tightness across the digestive zone

This texture is more than a physical anomaly—it is a **sensory signal** from the body's internal landscape. When you feel grit under your hands, you are touching the residue of what has not yet been processed or released. Supporting this area gently but intentionally helps restore both **physical function and emotional flow**.

Hollow Zones

Organ Removal, Digestive Disconnect

In reflexology, a **hollow or sunken area** in the arch of the foot is a significant marker—often subtle, but deeply revealing. These soft-tissue depressions commonly show up in zones corresponding to the **digestive tract**, **reproductive organs**, or **supportive detox systems** like the **liver and kidneys**. Rather than inflammation or congestion, hollow zones suggest an **absence of vitality** or **energetic disconnection** from the organ or system involved.

What a Hollow Zone Feels Like

To the practitioner:

- Noticeably **sunken or indented** compared to surrounding tissue
- Feels **cooler**, **less responsive**, or **flatter**
- May feel **"empty"** or energetically quiet when touched

To the client:

- May not register as painful—more often a "numb" or **dull zone**
- Clients may feel surprised by the lack of sensation or "hollowness"
- Some feel a **sense of detachment or dissociation** when the area is worked

What It May Indicate

1. Organ Removal

- Hysterectomy, gallbladder removal, appendectomy, etc.
- The body reflects the **loss of organ energy** in the corresponding reflex zone
- Can remain hollow years after surgery unless energetically addressed

2. Energetic Disconnect

- Client may **disassociate** from that body part due to trauma, grief, or shame
- Often found in cases of **sexual trauma**, **reproductive grief**, or **digestive fear**
- May reflect a **"shutdown"** in the enteric nervous system (gut-brain disconnection)

3. Long-term Depletion

- Chronic fatigue, burnout, or adrenal exhaustion
- Poor absorption and assimilation (especially if in small intestine zone)
- Emotional stagnation or years of **ignoring gut instincts**

Common Zones for Hollow Areas

- **Medial arch (inner foot):** Stomach, pancreas, liver, kidneys
- **Central arch:** Small intestine, absorption
- **Lateral arch (outer foot):** Colon, adrenals
- **Inner heel:** Uterus, ovaries, or prostate (especially post-surgery)

Emotional and Energetic Implications

- Digestive hollows often link with **not being able to "digest" life's experiences**
- Reproductive hollows may reflect **loss, grief, or unresolved trauma**
- Clients may use phrases like:
    - "I feel empty inside."
    - "I've never been the same since the surgery."
    - "I don't trust my gut anymore."

How to Support Hollow Zones

During the Reflexology Session:

- Use **gentle, nurturing pressure**—do not overstimulate
- Apply **Reiki** or energy healing to reconnect the zone
- Focus on **supportive, circular motions** to reawaken flow
- Combine with breathwork: encourage the client to **inhale into the zone**

Post-Session Support:

- **Energetic healing**: Chakra balancing, especially solar plexus and sacral
- **Emotional integration**: Somatic therapy, journaling, or trauma-informed practices
- **Nutritional rebuilding**: Iron, B12, adaptogens, and digestive bitters
- **Affirmations** for reconnection:
  "I honor my gut."
  "My body is whole, even in transition."
  "I welcome energy back to the parts of me that feel empty."

Client Confirmations

Clients with hollow digestive or reproductive reflexes often share:

- "I had that organ removed."
- "I haven't felt connected to that part of my body since the surgery."
- "I feel numb there—not just physically, but emotionally."
- "That's exactly where I feel most drained."

Practitioner Note

Hollow zones aren't always about absence—they can be **invitations for reconnection**. When approached with awareness, compassion, and curiosity, these quiet spaces often hold the greatest potential for healing.

Puffy Arch

Food Sensitivities, Inflammation

A **puffy or swollen arch** in reflexology is one of the most common and telling signs of internal stress in the **digestive system**, particularly when it relates to **inflammation**, **food sensitivities**, or **gut congestion**. Unlike a gritty or hollow zone, puffiness indicates a **build-up**—whether of fluids, unprocessed emotions, toxins, or poorly digested food and nutrients.

What a Puffy Arch Feels Like

To the practitioner:

- Feels **thick, spongy, or boggy** under the fingers
- May have **blunted contours**—the foot's shape seems less defined
- Can feel **cool or damp**, sometimes with a mild stickiness
- Pressing into the area may leave a faint **indent (edema)**

To the client:

- They may feel **tenderness** or **soreness** when touched
- Often report "bloated feet" or heaviness, especially after meals or in the evening
- Some may say they "hold tension in their gut" or are "sensitive to everything they eat"

What It May Indicate

1. Food Sensitivities or Intolerances

- Common with gluten, dairy, sugar, processed foods
- Puffy arch reflects **immune activation** in the gut wall or small intestine
- Can also correlate with **leaky gut syndrome** or microbiome imbalance

2. Systemic Inflammation

- Seen in clients with autoimmune conditions (IBS, Crohn's, Celiac)
- Generalized puffiness may indicate liver congestion and **poor detox capacity**
- Tied to poor lymphatic drainage, especially if arch puffiness extends toward the ankle

3. Digestive Stagnation

- Weak stomach acid or sluggish digestion
- Inability to break down food → fermentation → bloating → energetic congestion
- Puffy arch often corresponds with **fatigue, brain fog,** and **sluggish bowels**

Common Zones of Arch Puffiness

- **Central arch (small intestine):** Most common site of puffiness from food issues
- **Medial arch (stomach/pancreas):** Tied to sugar and carbohydrate overload
- **Outer arch (colon/adrenals):** Puffiness may reflect overburdened elimination pathways

Emotional and Energetic Associations

- Clients may be **"holding on" emotionally or mentally**—to old beliefs, relationships, or habits
- Food sensitivities often correspond with an **inability to "digest life"** or boundaries being crossed
- Common emotional themes:
  - "I don't feel nourished."
  - "I'm sensitive to everything."
  - "My body turns against me."

How to Support Puffy Arch Zones

During the Reflexology Session:

- Use **gentle lymphatic strokes**, moving toward drainage zones (heel and inner ankle)
- Add **circular stimulation** to stimulate digestion and flow
- Combine with **abdominal reflex zones** for improved motility
- Consider using **essential oils** (e.g., ginger, fennel, peppermint diluted in oil)

Post-Session Support:

- **Elimination diet** or sensitivity testing with a practitioner
- **Anti-inflammatory herbs and teas:** turmeric, ginger, chamomile
- **Rebounding or walking** to stimulate lymph and circulation
- **Castor oil packs** on the abdomen for liver and gut support
- **Probiotic and prebiotic foods** to repair gut flora
- Emotional self-inquiry: *"What am I struggling to digest?"*

Client Confirmations

Clients with puffy arches have often shared:

- "I feel bloated all the time."
- "My stomach is always upset when I eat gluten or dairy."
- "I'm always inflamed, and no one can figure out why."
- "My feet swell by the end of the day—especially after eating certain foods."

Practitioner Tip

Puffiness in the arch is often one of the **first signs** the body gives before more serious gut issues arise. When you notice it, **educate the client gently**—these are not random sensitivities, but messages from their body calling for deeper nourishment and attention.

Adrenal Burnout Signs

The **adrenal reflex zones** are located near the **upper medial arch**, just beneath the ball of the foot and slightly toward the inner edge. These tiny glands—despite their small size—play a **massive role** in our energy regulation, stress response, and overall hormonal balance.

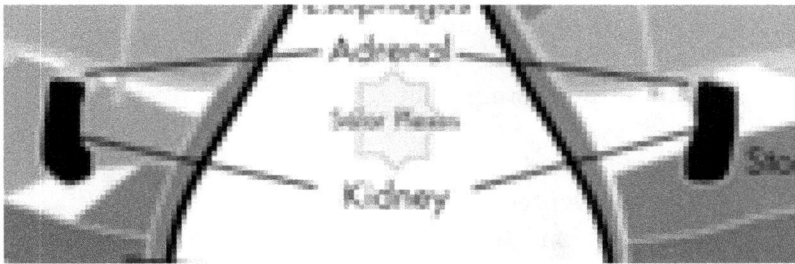

When the adrenals are overworked or depleted, their corresponding zones on the feet often show clear and tangible signs—both **physical** and **energetic**—that something is out of balance.

What It Feels Like in the Feet

To the practitioner:

- A **tight, rigid, or ropey texture** in the adrenal area
- May feel like a **thin tendon band** running vertically through the upper arch
- Occasionally **tender or reactive** with even light pressure
- Sometimes, this zone feels **shallow or sunken**—like the energy there has "collapsed"

To the client:

- May flinch or pull away slightly when the area is touched
- Some describe the pressure as "hitting a nerve" or "feeling raw"
- Clients often sigh, yawn, or take a deep breath when the area is released—indicating **nervous system reset**

What It May Indicate

1. Adrenal Fatigue or Burnout

- Result of long-term stress, poor sleep, or unresolved trauma
- Reflex zone may feel either **over-tense** (hypervigilance) or **sunken/depleted** (burnout)
- May correspond with **thyroid imbalance**, as the HPA axis is impacted

2. Chronic Fatigue or Wired-but-Tired States

- Reflex feels "hollow and tight"—a contradiction that reflects internal stress
- Clients often present with **daytime exhaustion** but difficulty sleeping
- May report craving salt or stimulants like caffeine or sugar

3. Overdrive/Control Personality Patterns

- Adrenal tension is often seen in high-functioning clients with **perfectionism, overwork, or chronic 'doing'**
- Emotionally, this zone can reflect a deep **inability to rest or receive**
- Phrase often heard: *"I'm fine. I'm just tired."*

Emotional and Energetic Correlations

- Over-control, fear of letting go
- Always "on," hyper-responsible, rarely asks for help
- Clients may say:
    - "I never stop."
    - "I feel like I'm running on fumes."
    - "I can't relax, even when I try."

How to Support Adrenal Zones

During Reflexology:

- Use **slow, steady, reassuring pressure**
- Combine with **solar plexus and diaphragm reflexes** to downshift nervous system
- Gentle circular motion or light pulsing can stimulate **rest and repair mode**
- Support with **heart and kidney reflexes**, as they often co-present with adrenal issues

After the Session:

- Recommend grounding practices (nature walks, earthing, journaling)
- Supportive nutrition: vitamin C, magnesium, adaptogens (ashwagandha, rhodiola)
- Hydration with electrolytes (especially Himalayan salt or trace minerals)
- Prioritize **rest without stimulation** (screens, to-do lists, etc.)
- Encourage breathwork or gentle yin-style movement (Tai Chi, restorative yoga)

Client Confirmations

Clients with adrenal tension zones have often shared:

- "That spot was tender—I feel that tension every day."
- "I've been going through a lot lately but I don't show it."
- "I'm so tired… but I can't seem to rest."
- "It's like my body is tired, but my brain won't shut off."

Practitioner Insight

The adrenal zones are **small but powerful storytellers**. When you work these reflexes with **compassion and awareness**, you often become the first person to help a client understand that exhaustion isn't weakness—it's a message. A call to slow down, soften, and start healing.

High vs. Flat Arches and What They Tell You

The **structure of the arch**—whether high, flat, or balanced—is more than just a biomechanical feature. In reflexology and energy medicine, the shape of the arch often reflects deep-seated **postural patterns, energetic tendencies, and emotional coping mechanisms**.

High Arches (Elevated, Rigid Footbeds)

Physical Observations:

- A pronounced lift in the midfoot
- Often accompanied by **tight calf muscles**, **rigid toes**, or **heel instability**
- Foot may appear narrow or overly curved

What It May Indicate:

- **Tension in the spine**—especially thoracic and lumbar areas
- **Adrenal overactivity** or chronic sympathetic dominance ("fight or flight")
- A tendency to **hold stress internally**—energy doesn't ground easily
- Often found in **perfectionists, over-achievers, or those who carry the world on their shoulders**

Emotional/Energetic Patterns:

- High arches suggest a **"lifted" or guarded stance**—as if the person is always bracing or preparing

- Energetically, this can symbolize a **lack of support or difficulty receiving**
- These clients may have difficulty letting go, trusting, or softening
- Disconnection from the Earth element—tendency to "live in the head"

Reflex Insights:

- Adrenal reflexes are often **tight or overactive**
- Digestive reflexes may feel **hollow** or **compacted**
- Foot may feel **tense or resistant to pressure**

Flat Arches (Collapsed or Fallen Arches)

Physical Observations:

- Minimal curvature in the midfoot
- Foot appears wide or spread out
- Ankles may roll inward (overpronation), leading to **knee/hip misalignment**

What It May Indicate:

- **Weak or depleted postural muscles**—especially in the core and lower back
- **Digestive sluggishness** or poor absorption (Earth and Water element deficiency)
- Often found in individuals with **chronic fatigue, grief, or depression**
- Tendency to **carry weight emotionally** or feel energetically "heavy"

Emotional/Energetic Patterns:

- Flat arches often indicate a person who feels **weighed down** or energetically "flattened"

- May symbolize **emotional overwhelm, responsibility overload**, or a sense of defeat
- In some cases, it can also show **over-grounding**—a person who is stuck, stagnant, or energetically compressed

Reflex Insights:

- Digestive and adrenal zones often feel **sluggish, mushy, or cold**
- Solar plexus area may be **blocked or underactive**
- Arch may hold **toxicity** or **gritty buildup** (especially in kidney/colon zones)

What Clients Often Say

High arch clients:

- "I can't relax—even when I try."
- "I hold everything in. I've always been the strong one."
- "My feet always cramp or feel tight."

Flat arch clients:

- "I feel tired all the time."
- "It's like I've lost my bounce."
- "My feet feel heavy and ache by the end of the day."

Practitioner Support Tips

For high arches:

- Use slow, grounding techniques—pressure into the arch can be deeply calming
- Focus on **solar plexus, adrenal, and kidney zones**
- Recommend grounding practices: barefoot walking, weighted blankets, slow movement

For flat arches:

- Stimulate circulation with **firm, uplifting strokes**
- Focus on **digestive and elimination reflexes**
- Offer support tools: Epsom foot soaks, breathwork, postural exercises, adrenal tonics

The shape of the arch reflects how a person **stands in life**—both literally and symbolically. High arches often reveal those who are "always on," holding themselves together with tension. Flat arches, on the other hand, may reflect those who've been carrying too much for too long and are in need of restoration. In reflexology, **how the foot holds itself** tells you as much as what lies beneath your hands.

Chapter 7: The Heel – Reproductive, Elimination, and Grounding Zones

Heel Calluses

IBS, Constipation, Pelvic Tension

The **heel area** of the foot is energetically and reflexively linked to **elimination, lower back, sacrum, and pelvic organs**. When thick, dry, or hardened skin forms in this region, it often signals more than just mechanical wear—it can be a **reflexive imprint of internal strain** or unresolved emotional holding in the lower body.

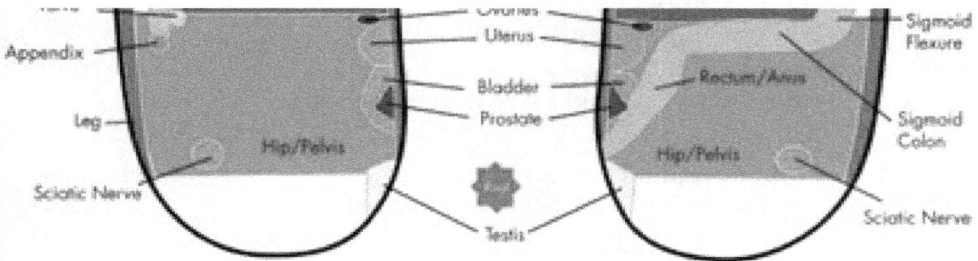

What Heel Calluses Look Like

- Dry, cracked, or thickened skin at the base or sides of the heel
- Often yellowish or gray in tone
- May extend into the outer edge or rise slightly onto the arch

What They May Indicate

1. Digestive & Elimination Imbalance

- **IBS, chronic constipation**, or irregular bowel habits
- Sluggish **colon reflex zones** often manifest as hardened tissue here
- Indicates the body's difficulty in **releasing waste**, both physically and energetically

2. Pelvic Floor Tension

- Emotional or physical trauma stored in the **sacral area**, such as:
    o Past sexual trauma
    o Chronic pelvic pain
    o Reproductive organ tension (e.g., endometriosis, fibroids)
- Callus buildup may indicate **energetic bracing**—the body holding in protection

3. Grounding & Root Chakra Disconnection

- Disconnection from **Earth energy** or a feeling of being "unrooted"
- May suggest a history of **survival-based stress**, insecurity, or fear
- Clients often feel emotionally unsupported or "on edge" without knowing why

Client Confirmations

- Clients with heel calluses often report:
  - Ongoing **bowel concerns** (especially stress-induced IBS)
  - Lower back tightness or chronic hip tension
  - Repressed emotions tied to safety, security, or past trauma
  - Fatigue that feels "heavier than tiredness"—a **draining weight in the body**

Supportive Approaches

Physical Therapies:

- **Exfoliating soaks** with Epsom salt, clay, or castor oil
- Reflexology work on **colon, sciatic, and pelvic reflexes**
- Gentle **pelvic floor release** or referrals for somatic pelvic therapy
- **Stretching routines** for lower back, hips, and psoas

Energetic Support:

- Root chakra healing: grounding meditations, red gemstones (e.g., garnet, red jasper)
- **Breathwork focused on exhalation** (release-oriented breathing)
- Journaling prompts:
  - "Where do I feel stuck or blocked in life?"
  - "What do I need to feel safe letting go of?"
  - "What am I carrying that isn't mine?"

Nutritional & Detox Support:

- Fiber-rich diet with hydration to ease bowel strain
- Herbal allies: **tripahala, psyllium, slippery elm** for bowel regulation

- Liver-supporting teas (e.g., dandelion root) if toxicity is suspected

Visual & Energetic Observation

Heel calluses can be read like **emotional fossils**—compressed remnants of resistance, protection, and holding. Often, they reflect **years of internalized tension**, especially in those who struggle to let go physically or emotionally.

Puffy Around Ankle

Sciatic Nerve Stress, Ovary/Testicle Zones

Swelling or puffiness around the **inner and outer ankles** can offer powerful insight into the health of the **pelvis, reproductive system, and lower spine**, especially the **sciatic nerve and sacral reflex zones**. The ankles act as energetic portals that mirror how freely life force energy flows through the base of the body.

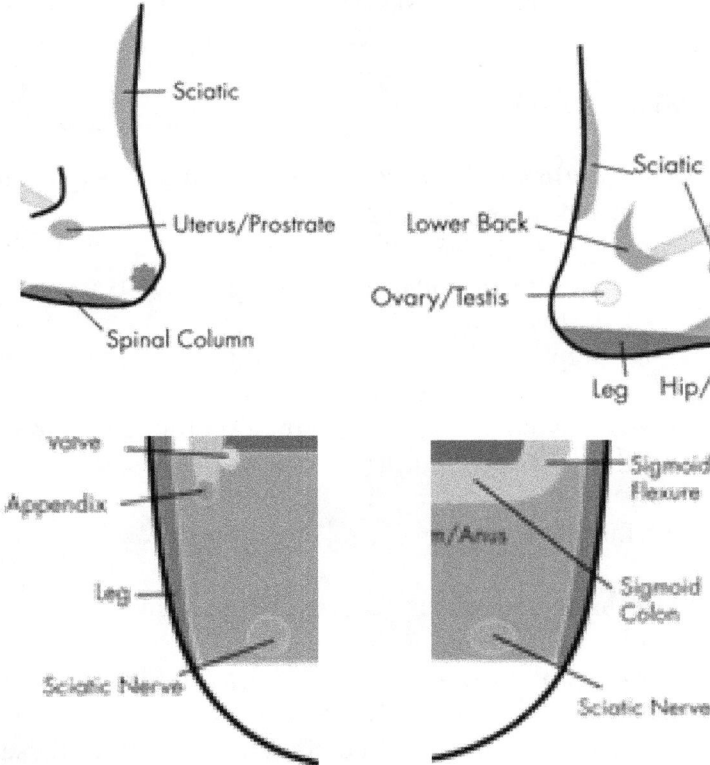

What Puffy Ankles Suggest

1. Sciatic Nerve Stress

- The outer ankle area aligns with the **sciatic nerve reflex,** running down the leg from the sacral spine.
- Puffiness may indicate:
    - **Compression or inflammation** of the sciatic nerve
    - Overuse from standing, poor posture, or imbalanced gait
    - Lumbar spine misalignment or tight piriformis/glute muscles
- Clients may report lower back pain, hip discomfort, or leg numbness/tingling.

2. Ovary/Testicle Reflex Stress

- **Inner ankle puffiness** corresponds with the **ovaries (in women)** or **testes (in men).**
- Swelling here can reflect:
    - Hormonal imbalance (PMS, menopause, low testosterone)
    - Reproductive organ congestion or inflammation
    - Fertility issues, cysts, or past trauma
- Clients may not always be aware of reproductive strain until this is pointed out.

Other Contributing Factors

- **Lymphatic stagnation** (especially post-illness or with sluggish elimination)
- **Kidney and adrenal strain** (may lead to lower leg swelling)
- Footwear that impedes circulation or compresses these reflex zones

- **Energetic congestion** from emotional holding in the pelvis

Client Confirmations

Clients with puffy ankles often validate:

- **Sciatic pain or nerve discomfort**, especially with a history of sitting long hours
- Past or current **ovarian/testicular issues**, including surgeries, fertility struggles, or sexual trauma
- Sensations of **pressure, heaviness, or fullness** in the lower abdomen
- Unexpected **emotional releases** when these zones are worked on

Supportive Approaches

Physical Therapies:

- Reflexology techniques for **sciatic nerve relief** and **reproductive organs**
- Stretching: gentle **hip openers, piriformis release, spinal elongation**
- Manual lymphatic drainage or **ankle rotation exercises**
- Warm foot soaks with **magnesium** to reduce swelling

Energetic & Emotional Support:

- Sacral chakra balancing through Reiki, breathwork, or pelvic journaling
- Visualization: imagine **fluid clearing** from the ankles downward into the Earth
- Journaling prompts:
  - "Where am I holding too tightly?"
  - "What part of me feels unsupported?"

- o "What am I ready to release from my lower body?"

Nutritional/Herbal Aids:

- Hydration and electrolyte balance
- Herbs that support hormonal balance and lymphatic flow (e.g., red clover, burdock, nettle)
- Anti-inflammatory diet to support circulation and detox

Practitioner Tips

- **Note symmetry**: bilateral puffiness often indicates systemic lymph or kidney issues, while one-sided puffiness may point to localized structural or reproductive concerns.
- Check the **texture**: soft/fluid puffiness indicates lymph; harder swelling may be fibrotic or chronic tension.

Dryness, Cracking, and Grounding Energy Issues

The **heels** represent our connection to the Earth—our **grounding zone**. When the skin here becomes dry, cracked, or excessively callused, it often reflects more than just lack of moisture. These are signs that **root-level imbalance** is present, and the body is sending signals about stability, security, and basic survival energy.

What Dry, Cracked Heels Reveal

1. Grounding Deficiency

- The **heels correspond to the root chakra** (Muladhara), associated with:
  o Feeling safe and supported
  o Financial or physical security
  o Home, tribe, and belonging
- Chronic dryness or cracking often reflects **ungrounded energy**—a person may be:
  o Overthinking or "in their head" too much
  o Struggling with anxiety, instability, or constant change
  o Lacking time in nature or physical movement

2. Kidney/Adrenal Imbalance

- Cracked heels may signal **adrenal fatigue**, dehydration, or kidney stress—often related to:
  o Long-term stress or burnout
  o Fear-based responses (fight-or-flight stuck "on")
  o Nutrient depletion (especially minerals)

3. Structural and Postural Load

- The heels bear the **entire body's weight**—they may crack when:
    - The individual is carrying too much "pressure"
    - Standing, caregiving, or holding responsibility for others
    - Shoes don't support natural gait or shock absorption

Energetic Themes

- **Cracks** = "Fractures" in personal foundation, possibly from past trauma or instability
- **Dryness** = Withheld nourishment, emotional depletion, lack of joy or pleasure
- **Hardness** = Armor from fear, distrust, or suppressed anger

Client Confirmations

Clients with dry, cracked heels often admit to:

- **Chronic stress or anxiety**
- Feeling **ungrounded, overwhelmed, or unsupported**
- Past **financial struggles, family instability**, or burnout
- A sense of being "cut off" from their body or emotions

Supportive Approaches

Physical Therapies:

- Exfoliating scrubs and **moisturizing foot masks**
- Reflexology or **root chakra energy balancing**
- Gentle massage to restore warmth and circulation
- Supportive footwear to improve heel strike cushioning

Energetic Support:

- **Grounding meditations** or barefoot walking in nature
- Root chakra affirmations:
  "I am safe." "I am supported." "I belong."
- Visualization: red energy flowing up from the Earth into the heels and legs

Topical & Internal Support:

- Oils: Castor, shea butter, coconut with essential oils like frankincense or myrrh
- Herbal support: **Nettle, ashwagandha, licorice root** for adrenal/grounding help
- Hydration and **electrolyte balance** (especially magnesium)

Practitioner Tips

- **Assess the location and depth** of cracking—deep central fissures may indicate chronic root stress, while surface dryness may be more environmental.
- Invite clients to **reconnect to their physical body** with grounding rituals and restorative rest.

Signs of Reproductive Trauma or Hormone Depletion

The inner and outer heel—especially around the **ankle bone, heel edge, and Achilles tendon**—corresponds to the **reproductive organs** in reflexology. For women, this includes the **ovaries, uterus, and fallopian tubes**; for men, the **testicles and prostate**. These zones can reveal a remarkable amount about a person's **hormonal health, reproductive history**, and **energetic imprint of trauma**.

What the Heels Can Reveal About Reproductive Health

1. Puffiness or Swelling Around the Inner Ankle

- Often found in clients with:
    - **Menstrual issues**, such as irregular periods or endometriosis
    - **Fertility struggles** or hormonal imbalances (low progesterone or estrogen dominance)
    - **Polycystic ovarian syndrome (PCOS)**
    - **Testicular inflammation** or past infection in male clients

2. Tenderness or Rigidity

- Common in clients with past:
    - **Surgical interventions** (e.g., hysterectomy, vasectomy, C-section, abortion)
    - **Sexual trauma or abuse**

- o **Shame, grief, or disconnection** from their reproductive system
- The tissue may feel **hard, unresponsive, or emotionally guarded**

3. Hollow or Sunken Zones

- Suggestive of:
  - o **Removed organs** (e.g., uterus, ovary, testicle)
  - o **Energetic depletion** from years of hormonal or emotional strain
  - o **Suppressed libido** or disconnection from sensuality and creativity
- Some clients describe this as "numbness" or an inability to feel that part of their body

4. Gritty Texture

- Reflects toxic buildup or **poor lymphatic drainage** around the pelvic area
- Common in:
  - o Long-term **birth control use**
  - o **Hormone replacement therapy**
  - o **Estrogen dominance** or liver sluggishness
  - o **Stored trauma** in the womb/prostate

Emotional & Energetic Themes

- **Left heel (feminine side)**: Tied to mothering energy, receiving, intuition, and inner cycles
- **Right heel (masculine side)**: Reflects doing, providing, control, and external expression

Common emotional patterns:

- Shame, guilt, or grief around reproduction or sexuality

- Suppressed creativity or loss of identity through reproductive illness
- Burnout from caregiving roles, miscarriage, or loss

Client Confirmations

Clients with these signs often report:

- **Hysterectomy**, tubal ligation, or **IVF** struggles
- Painful periods, irregular cycles, or **early menopause**
- Low libido, hormonal migraines, or mood swings
- Past **sexual trauma** that they may not have disclosed before

Supportive Practices

Physical Interventions:

- **Reflexology protocols** for endocrine and pelvic balance
- Pelvic steaming (yoni steams) with herbs like **mugwort, rose, lavender**
- **Castor oil packs** on the lower abdomen or around the heel zone

Hormonal Support:

- Adaptogens like **maca, ashwagandha, vitex**
- Nutritional support with **omega-3s, B-vitamins, magnesium, and zinc**
- Detoxification pathways (especially liver and lymph)

Energetic Healing:

- Reiki or chakra balancing focused on the **sacral chakra**
- Visualization: reconnecting to the womb/testicles as creative, sacred centers

- Journaling prompts:
  "What do I still carry in my body from the past?"
  "What would healing feel like for my creative/reproductive self?"

Chapter 8: Dorsal Foot – The Spine, Shoulders, and Emotional Armor

Tight or Bony Shoulder Ridge

The **dorsal (top) surface of the foot**, just below the base of the toes, represents the **shoulder and upper back** reflex zones in reflexology. This area is often one of the most **structurally and emotionally revealing regions** of the foot, especially when it presents as **tight, bony, or rigid**.

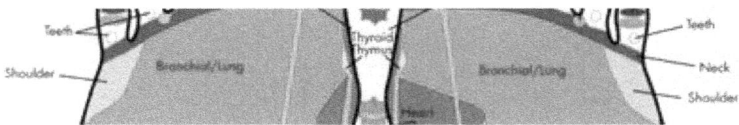

What Is the Shoulder Ridge?

The **shoulder ridge** runs horizontally across the top of the foot, just beneath the metatarsal heads (ball of the foot area). It mirrors the **physical shoulder girdle** and **upper trapezius**, and energetically it reflects the burdens and responsibilities a person is "carrying" in life.

Signs to Observe

1. Bony Prominence or Knobs

- Often felt as small, hard protrusions under the skin
- Indicates:
    - o **Chronic shoulder tension** (often in desk workers, hairstylists, or massage therapists)
    - o **Poor posture**, especially forward-head or rounded-shoulder posture
    - o Possible **frozen shoulder**, rotator cuff injury, or previous trauma

2. Rigidity or Inflexibility

- Tissue feels stiff, resistant, or like it lacks elasticity
- Associated with:
    - o **Control issues** or fear of letting go
    - o Long-held **stress or grief** stored in the upper back
    - o Clients who tend to "hold it all together" or carry others' emotional weight

3. Tightness or Ropey Texture

- Feels like tight bands or sinewy cords under the skin
- Common in clients who:
    - o Feel **emotionally burdened**
    - o Are navigating **stressful relationships** or **caretaking roles**
    - o Have a history of **emotional suppression**, particularly of anger or grief

Emotional Patterns and Symbolism

The shoulder zone is often where people "store" emotional weight—particularly:

- **Unexpressed emotions**
- **Caretaking burdens**
- **Responsibility overload**
- **Perfectionism** or always "being strong"

Clients with this tension may describe:

- Feeling like they "can't put it down"
- Chronic neck or shoulder pain, even without injury
- Dreams of flying, falling, or carrying heavy loads

Client Confirmations

In sessions, clients often validate:

- "That's exactly where I carry my tension."
- "I've had frozen shoulder on that side."
- "I never realized how heavy everything feels until now."

Some even report **emotional release** (tears, deep exhales, spontaneous memories) when this area is worked with gentleness and intention.

Supportive Techniques

Manual Support

- Focused thumb walking or circular motion on the dorsal shoulder ridge
- Soften with warm compresses or gentle fascial work before deeper pressure

Energetic & Emotional Support

- Chakra clearing, especially **heart and throat**
- Journaling prompt:
  "Whose weight am I carrying that isn't mine to hold?"
- Emotional clearing exercises or auric release techniques
- Flower essences (e.g., Elm for overwhelm, Oak for endurance fatigue)

Postural & Lifestyle Suggestions

- Encourage awareness of posture, shoulder mobility, and breathwork
- Recommend stretching (e.g., eagle arms, shoulder rolls, doorway chest openers)
- Cross-referral to RMT, chiropractor, or yoga therapist when appropriate

Calluses on Dorsal Toes

Top of Toes

Indicators of Dental Stress & Emotional Strain

Calluses that form on the **dorsal (top) side of the toes**, particularly near the knuckles or joints, are often **overlooked** in traditional reflexology—but they carry potent diagnostic and energetic clues. These dorsal toe calluses are not just the result of poor footwear. They frequently correlate with **dental trauma, jaw misalignment, and deep-seated emotional holding**, especially in the **throat, jaw, and mind-body communication pathways**.

What to Look For

- **Thickened skin** across the top of one or more toes (especially 1st and 2nd toes)
- **Localized dryness, ridging, or cracked skin**
- Sometimes paired with **underlying toe curvature or overlapping**

What It May Indicate

Dental/Orthodontic Stress

- Reflexology and energetic mapping correlate dorsal toe regions (especially the 1st and 2nd toes) with the **jaw, teeth, TMJ (temporomandibular joint), and upper neck**.
- Dorsal toe calluses are commonly found in people with:
  - **Extensive dental work** (fillings, extractions, root canals)

- o **Braces or retainers**, especially from childhood
- o **Chronic jaw tension or clenching**
- o **Night grinding (bruxism)** or stress-related jaw pain

Practitioner insight:

Clients with these calluses often report:

"I've always had jaw tension," or "I clench my teeth at night."

Emotional Holding in the Mouth & Expression

- The top of the toes—particularly the big toe—also reflects **mental strain and emotional inhibition**.
- Calluses here can indicate:
  - o **Suppressed communication** (not speaking truth, fear of confrontation)
  - o **Overthinking or internalized stress**
  - o **Old emotional trauma stored in the body**, especially grief or shame that was never expressed

"This callus is where you've walked through life with your words held back."

Common Patterns by Toe:

- **Big toe (1st):** TMJ, dental trauma, unspoken truths, grief held in the throat
- **2nd toe:** Analytical overdrive, excessive mental chatter, perfectionism
- **3rd toe:** Self-criticism, frustration, stuck decision-making
- **4th/5th toes:** Body-image tension, fear of vulnerability, emotional withdrawal

Support Options

Physical Support

- Soothing foot soaks with Epsom salts and essential oils (lavender, myrrh, frankincense)
- Gentle exfoliation and castor oil packs
- Craniosacral therapy or TMJ-specific bodywork
- Dental consultation if significant mouth/jaw symptoms persist

Emotional & Energetic Release

- Reiki or auric field clearing around throat and jaw chakras
- Guided journaling:
  - *"What do I need to say that I've been holding back?"*
  - *"What tension am I still chewing on?"*
- Breathwork with a focus on the **throat and jaw release**

Flower Essences

- **Blue Vervain**: For tension and control
- **Mimulus**: For fear of expressing oneself
- **Chicory or Pine**: For emotional guilt and withheld affection

In Practice: **Clients often experience significant** emotional insights or releases **when this area is gently explored. Some report that after sessions:**

- Dreams resurface around **childhood orthodontic trauma**
- Their **voice feels stronger** or **jaw tension decreases**
- Emotions like **grief or frustration** bubble up for healing

Spine Zone Distortions and Posture Reading

Dorsal Foot + Medial Arch

How the Feet Mirror the Spine and Musculoskeletal Alignment

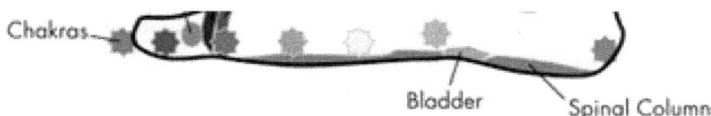

Chakras — ... — Bladder — Spinal Column

The feet tell the story of your **posture, spinal tension, and alignment**—sometimes more clearly than the back itself. In reflexology, the **inner (medial) edge of the foot** reflects the **entire spinal column**, from the cervical vertebrae near the big toe to the sacrum near the heel. The **dorsal (top) foot** also gives clues about muscular tension, shoulder positioning, and overall gait compensation.

What to Look For:

- Irregularities or bulges along the **medial arch**
- Collapsed or overly rigid inner foot
- Dorsal foot bony ridges, especially near metatarsals
- Pressure differences between feet (one arch higher or flatter)

Spinal Map on the Foot (Medial Side)

- **Big toe base = Cervical spine (neck)**
- **Ball of foot = Thoracic spine (upper/mid-back)**
- **Arch = Lumbar spine (low back)**
- **Heel = Sacrum and coccyx (tailbone)**

Common Distortions and Their Meanings:

Bulging or Raised Areas (Hypertonicity)

- May indicate muscle overuse, chronic stress, or **vertebral misalignment**
- Often seen in those who **carry others emotionally or physically**
- Related symptoms: **Neck stiffness, headaches, upper back tension**

Sunken or Flattened Zones (Hypotonicity)

- Suggests **energy depletion** in spinal support systems
- May reflect **nervous system exhaustion** or poor postural engagement
- Related symptoms: **Fatigue, spinal collapse, poor core stability**

Sharp Ridges or Pain on Pressure

- Can indicate old **injuries, spinal compression, or herniation**
- Clients may confirm a **history of falls, accidents, or postural strain**

Asymmetry Between Left and Right

- One foot shows tension, the other weakness
- Often reflects **gait imbalances, scoliosis, or compensatory patterns**

- Also may suggest an **energetic imbalance between masculine and feminine polarities**

Postural Insights From the Feet:

- **Collapsed arch = adrenal fatigue or lumbar strain**
- **Tense, tight arch = rigidity, spinal guarding, suppressed emotions**
- **Thickened skin at heel edge = sacral holding, often sexual or reproductive tension**
- **Flat footedness = instability, emotional overwhelm, digestive energy depletion**

"The foot arch reflects your spine's story—its strength, its strain, and the weight you've carried."

Support Options:

Structural & Physical

- Chiropractic or osteopathic adjustments
- Core strengthening through yoga or Pilates
- Barefoot walking for realignment and proprioception
- Craniosacral therapy for nervous system recalibration

Energetic & Emotional

- Reiki over the spine and root chakra
- Guided body scans or breathwork for postural release
- Journaling prompt:
  "Where am I carrying weight that isn't mine?"
  "What support do I need to stand tall again?"

In Session Observation Tip:

If you trace your thumb along the medial arch and feel bumps, hollows, or tenderness, pause and ask:

"Do you ever experience tension or discomfort in your lower back/upper spine/neck?"

You'll be surprised how often clients respond:

"Yes! How did you know that?"

Skin Tone, Sensitivity, and Fascia Tension

What the Dorsal Foot Reveals

The **dorsal (top) side of the foot** is more than a bony structure with tendons—it's a **sensitive canvas** that reflects **nervous system tone**, **circulatory health**, and **emotional tension stored in the fascia**. Changes in skin color, touch sensitivity, and fascial tension in this area can point to systemic imbalances and long-held emotional patterns.

What to Look For:

1. Skin Tone Variations

- **Pale or bluish tone:** May indicate poor **circulation, anemia**, or **nervous system fatigue**
- **Redness or flushed tone:** Suggests **acute stress**, inflammation, or **sympathetic overdrive**
- **Blotchy/mottled skin:** Linked to **emotional instability**, anxiety, or systemic vascular irregularities
- **Glossy/thin skin:** Often seen in clients with **adrenal depletion** or long-term **burnout**
- **Yellow tint:** May relate to **liver toxicity** or poor lymphatic drainage

2. Sensitivity to Touch

- **Tender or hypersensitive areas** (especially over joints or tendons) often reflect:
  - **Inflamed fascia or tendons**
  - **Unprocessed emotional pain**

- o **Overstimulation of the nervous system**
- **Numbness or dull sensation** may signal:
  - o **Energetic shutdown**, past trauma, or neurological disconnection
  - o **Peripheral circulation issues** (especially in diabetic or post-surgical clients)

Client insight:

"It doesn't hurt, but I barely feel it there." → Signals numbness, energetic withdrawal

"That's too tender to touch!" → Often relates to emotional shock zones or recent stress

3. Fascial Tension (Top of Foot and Ankle Zone)

- **Tight cords or bands under skin** suggest:
  - o **Overuse**, especially in those who stand a lot or wear restrictive shoes
  - o Emotional holding in the **solar plexus or shoulder zones**
- **Restricted dorsiflexion (toes pulling back)** may point to:
  - o **Fear of forward movement** or feeling emotionally "stuck"
  - o Physical ankle instability or spinal/postural compensation

Energetically, fascial tension mirrors **resistance to change, emotional bracing**, or long-held grief.

Journaling Prompt:

"Where in my life am I holding tension that's no longer serving me?"

"What part of myself do I need to reconnect with?"

Interpretation Examples:

Observation	Possible Root Cause	Emotional Layer
Redness & tension on top of foot	Inflammation, tension in shoulders or upper spine	Emotional overload, suppressed frustration
Cool, pale skin & loss of tone	Weak circulation, adrenal fatigue	Lack of support, collapse under pressure
Overreactive sensitivity	Nervous system stress	Past trauma, fight-or-flight activation
Ropey fascial bands across tendons	Chronic overwork, postural strain	Bracing for emotional impact

Support Options:

- **Massage & fascial release:** Light traction, ankle circles, and myofascial work help loosen tension
- **Hydration & minerals:** Especially magnesium and electrolytes for fascia support
- **Energy healing or grounding techniques:** Restore awareness to numbed or disconnected zones
- **Foot soaks or castor oil packs:** Reduce inflammation and soften hardened tissue
- **Breathwork or tapping (EFT):** To release sympathetic overdrive and emotional rigidity

Chapter 9: Temperature, Texture & Circulation

Cold vs. Warm Areas – Energetic and Physical Insights

Temperature differences across the feet are among the **most reliable indicators** of both **circulatory health** and **energetic flow**. Cold or hot zones often appear **before medical symptoms** arise and are deeply connected to **nervous system activity**, **organ function**, and **emotional holding patterns**.

What Cold Areas Reveal:

Physical Insights:

- **Poor circulation**: Common in extremities, especially in the elderly or those with cardiovascular concerns.
- **Thyroid imbalance**: Particularly hypothyroidism; slow metabolism leads to cold hands and feet.
- **Adrenal fatigue**: When the body is depleted, blood flow may be prioritized to core organs, reducing peripheral warmth.
- **Blood sugar issues**: Insulin resistance or low blood sugar can affect capillary perfusion.

Energetic Insights:

- **Energetic withdrawal or shutdown** in the corresponding reflex zone
- **Disconnection or trauma**—often in zones where a client has emotionally "numbed out"
- **Root chakra imbalance**: Cold feet may indicate instability, fear, or survival stress.

Common Cold Zones:

- **Toes**: Brain fatigue, cognitive fog, anxiety
- **Heel**: Root issues, lower back fatigue, reproductive depletion
- **Outer edge**: Muscular or joint shutdown (hips, shoulders)

What Warm or Hot Areas Reveal:

Physical Insights:

- **Inflammation or infection** in the corresponding organ system
- **Stress-related overactivity**, especially in adrenal, digestive, or cardiovascular zones
- **Menopause/perimenopause**: Hot spots (especially on arches or balls of the feet) may show hormonal fluctuations

Energetic Insights:

- **Stored anger or irritation**—commonly felt in liver or gallbladder zones
- **Emotional reactivation**: A once-numb area beginning to "wake up" may feel hot or tingly
- **Solar plexus overload**: Stress, anxiety, control issues often show heat in the upper arch

Common Warm Zones:

- **Ball of foot**: Heart stress, adrenal overdrive
- **Arch**: Digestive inflammation, emotional overload
- **Ankles**: Hormonal or reproductive heat (e.g., ovulation, hot flashes)

Combined Clues: Hot & Cold Together

When one area is hot and another is cold, the body may be in **energetic conflict** or compensating between systems. For example:

- **Cold feet with hot arches** → adrenal fatigue + digestive hyperactivity
- **Warm heel with cold toes** → reproductive strain + cognitive depletion

Areas That Change Temperature During a Reflexology Session

—A Window into Energetic Shifts and Healing Response—

One of the most subtle yet telling signs during a reflexology session is the **change in temperature** across specific zones of the feet. These fluctuations are not random—they reflect real-time shifts in **nervous system activation**, **energy release**, and **circulatory changes** linked to the reflexes being worked.

What It Means When an Area Warms Up:

- **Energetic "thawing" or activation** – Often seen in areas that initially feel cold, tight, or unresponsive. As energy begins to flow, blood returns to the area and the tissues soften.

- **Nervous system engagement** – Warming can indicate that the body is moving from sympathetic (stress response) into parasympathetic (rest/heal) mode.
- **Emotional release** – Sometimes correlated with tearfulness, deep sighs, or a sense of "lightness" in clients.

Example: A cold heel that begins to warm during the session may reflect the release of root chakra tension or pelvic congestion.

What It Means When an Area Cools Down:

- **Energetic release or discharge** – An area that was "hot" due to inflammation, stress, or anger may cool as that energy clears.
- **Overstimulation** – If a zone cools and loses vitality, the area may have been worked too intensely or for too long.
- **Avoidance pattern** – In some cases, sudden cooling can reflect emotional shutdown or avoidance, especially if the client seems withdrawn or mentally distracted.

Example: The ball of the foot (heart/adrenal reflex) that starts warm but goes cool may suggest emotional overwhelm giving way to fatigue.

Shifting Zones: Interpreting Patterns

- **Warm → Cold → Warm**
  = Layered emotional release or energetic detox, especially in chronic pain zones.
- **Cold → Warm → Tingling**
  = Nerve reactivation or reconnection to sensation in previously numbed areas.

- **Sudden flush of heat**
  = A "breakthrough" moment—pay attention to body language or emotional cues.

Practitioner Tips for Tracking Temperature Changes:

Practice	Why It Matters
Light resting hand	Sense thermal shifts without influencing them
Begin session with a foot scan	Establish a temperature baseline
Check same zones post-session	Note changes and document patterns over time
Ask client subtle questions	"Does this feel different now?" vs. "Does this feel warmer?" (to avoid leading)

How to Support Sudden Temperature Shifts:

- **Cool compress or calming oils** if excess heat emerges
- **Extra grounding or energy sweeping** if a client becomes spacey after a zone goes cold
- **Slow, soothing integration strokes** when deep shifts are felt (especially with trauma zones)
- **Post-session rest or journaling** to allow integration of released emotional or energetic data

Practitioner Reflection Prompt:

"What area changed most during the session, and how did the client respond physically or emotionally when it did?"

Practitioner Tools & Tips:

Observation	Potential Action
Cold toes and outer edge	Check for shoulder/brain fatigue; encourage movement and circulation
Hot ball of foot	Gently soothe with cooling oils (lavender, chamomile); assess for heart/adrenal stress
Alternating hot/cold areas	Invite emotional dialogue; check for recent trauma or stress
Chronically cold zones	Energy healing, grounding work, thyroid/adrenal referrals

Support Strategies:

- **Hydrotherapy**: Alternating hot/cold foot baths to stimulate flow
- **Essential oils**: Ginger, cinnamon for cold; peppermint or eucalyptus for heat
- **Manual stimulation**: Reflexology, acupressure, or massage to awaken numb zones
- **Nutrition**: Iron, B12, adaptogens for cold; anti-inflammatory support for hot
- **Movement**: Rebounding, tai chi, or walking barefoot to improve energy flow

Journaling Prompt for Clients:

"Where in my life do I feel frozen or numb?
Where am I burning out or holding too much heat?"

Circulatory Issues, Thyroid Indicators, and Adrenal Stress in the Feet

The feet are rich in vascular, endocrine, and nervous system reflexes—making them powerful indicators of deeper systemic imbalances. Three common patterns often overlap in reflexology sessions: **poor circulation, thyroid dysfunction,** and **adrenal fatigue**. Here's how they present and what they can reveal:

Circulatory Issues

Common Signs:

- **Cold toes or feet** (even in warm environments)
- **Mottled or bluish skin tone**, especially on the soles
- **Slow skin rebound** when pressing the tissue
- **Thickened toenails** or **loss of hair** on toes (chronic signs)
- **Swelling around ankles or instep**

Associated Reflex Zones:

- Heart (ball of the left foot)
- Circulatory and lymphatic zones along the inner foot
- Kidney/adrenal and liver reflexes (which support blood filtration and volume)

Client Correlations:

- History of anemia, low blood pressure, diabetes, varicose veins
- Sedentary lifestyle or prolonged sitting
- Women over 50 (hormonal decline affecting vascular tone)

Support Suggestions:

- Warm foot soaks or alternating hot/cold compresses
- Circulation-boosting essential oils (rosemary, black pepper, ginger)
- Referral for cardiovascular checkups if persistent

Thyroid Indicators

Common Signs in Reflexology:

- **Persistent coldness**, especially in the toes and ball of the foot
- **Pale, dry, or flaky skin**, especially on heels and outer edges
- **Low muscle tone** or "spongy" feel in the arch
- **Toenail ridges or brittleness**

Reflex Zones:

- Thyroid: under the big toe pad (both feet)
- Parathyroid: medial corner of the big toe
- Pituitary: center of big toe tip (hormonal cascade connection)

Client Correlations:

- Fatigue, sluggish metabolism, depression, brain fog
- Known hypothyroid diagnosis or family history

- Menstrual irregularities or menopausal symptoms

Support Suggestions:

- Nutritional support (iodine-rich foods, selenium, adaptogens)
- Gentle neck/shoulder work (thyroid-throat chakra connection)
- Energy healing or Reiki to the thyroid and hormonal grid

Adrenal Stress

Common Signs:

- **Puffy arches** (especially medial side = kidney/adrenal reflexes)
- **Redness or heat in the center of the arch**
- **Tension bands** across the arch or instep
- **High arch structure** (linked to chronic sympathetic dominance)
- **Client reports of chronic fatigue or "wired but tired" feeling**

Reflex Zones:

- Adrenals: center of each arch
- Kidneys: slightly above adrenal reflex
- Solar plexus: center of diaphragm line (ball of foot)

Client Correlations:

- Chronic stress, burnout, sleep issues
- Caffeine or stimulant dependency
- Emotional fragility or irritability

Support Suggestions:

- Foot holds with deep diaphragmatic breathing
- Soothing techniques like warm compresses, lavender or vetiver oils
- Encourage clients to track energy cycles and rest appropriately

Interconnected Patterns

Many clients will show **overlap** in these categories. For example:

- **Cold, dry feet with high arches** → adrenal + thyroid combo
- **Swollen ankles + gritty arch texture** → circulation + elimination stress
- **Tender big toe pads + fatigue** → thyroid + hormonal imbalance

Practitioner Tip:

Always look at **color, texture, temperature, and tissue tone** together for a full picture. These systems are interrelated—and your hands may detect imbalances before clients are even aware of them.

Foot Sweating, Odor, and Their Holistic Meanings

Although often overlooked or dismissed as hygiene issues, **excessive foot sweating** and **persistent foot odor** can be important indicators of internal imbalances, energetic blockages, or emotional states. In reflexology and holistic practices, these signs offer insight into both the **physical state of the body** and the **emotional or energetic patterns** a person may be unconsciously holding.

Excessive Foot Sweating (Hyperhidrosis)

Physical Indicators:

- Overactive sympathetic nervous system ("fight or flight" dominance)
- Thyroid imbalance (especially hyperthyroidism)
- Hormonal fluctuations (adolescents, perimenopause, etc.)
- Blood sugar instability (hypoglycemia or early diabetes)
- Stress, anxiety, or panic patterns (even if unspoken)

Energetic/Emotional Insights:

- Emotional tension stored in the **solar plexus** or **adrenal zones** (center of the arch)
- Subconscious **fear of being seen, judged, or failing**
- Individuals who push through stress rather than pause or rest

Client Clues:

- Nervous personality or perfectionist tendencies
- "High achiever" who may burn out easily
- Reports of hands also sweating under stress

Reflex Zones to Focus On:

- Adrenal glands (center of arch)
- Diaphragm/solar plexus line (ball of foot)
- Pituitary and thyroid zones (big toe and pads)

Support Suggestions:

- Calming reflexology session with grounding oils (vetiver, patchouli)
- Breathwork to soothe the solar plexus
- Referral to TCM or naturopathic support for hormone balancing

Foot Odor (Bromhidrosis)

Physical Causes:

- Accumulated bacteria breaking down sweat (due to poor air flow or synthetic socks)
- Imbalanced gut flora or high toxic load
- Liver or kidney overload (inability to detox efficiently)
- Certain medications or high consumption of garlic/onions/spices

Energetic/Emotional Insights:

- **Liver-related emotions** such as **anger, frustration, or resentment** may "leak" through scent
- Clients who feel energetically "stuck," repressed, or overwhelmed

- Suppressed emotional grief or shame (especially if odor is sour or sharp)

Clues to Watch For:

- Odor that persists even with good hygiene
- Clients with digestive issues, bloating, or skin breakouts
- Irregular elimination or history of detox difficulty

Relevant Reflex Zones:

- Liver and gallbladder (right foot arch)
- Kidneys and colon (both arches and heels)
- Lymphatic zones (upper instep, between toes)

Support Suggestions:

- Dry brushing and foot scrubs with detoxifying herbs (rosemary, juniper)
- Reflexology sessions focused on liver, kidney, and lymph drainage
- Nutritional guidance (reduce processed foods, increase greens/water)

Energetic Meaning of Moisture and Scent in the Feet

- **Excessive moisture** = overstimulation, emotional discharge, or sympathetic overdrive
- **Dry but smelly feet** = trapped toxins, lymph stagnation, or mental overwhelm
- **Cold and wet feet** = possible kidney or adrenal depletion
- **Sour/sweaty odor** = unresolved stress or liver overload
- **Musky odor** = hormonal changes or endocrine disturbance

Practitioner Considerations:

- Avoid making clients feel self-conscious—approach with neutrality and curiosity.
- Use "I've noticed some moisture/tension here—do you tend to run warm or feel stressed?"
- If a client apologizes, reassure them that their body is simply **communicating**.

Chapter 10: Case-Based Signs & Confirmations

Client Case Examples

(Fictionalized but Based on Real Patterns)

To help bring the signs to life, here are a few fictionalized examples drawn from actual sessions over the years. These stories show how reflexology signs—like puffiness, hollows, and calluses—often correlate with real-life health conditions or emotional stressors.

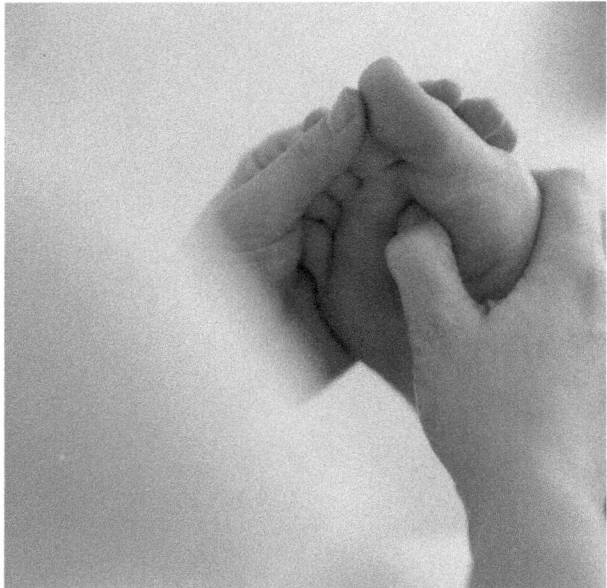

Each case is simplified and anonymized but offers insight into how these signs were interpreted, how the client responded, and what actions followed.

Case 1: Puffy Pads & Silent Sinuses

Client: *"Mary," a 42-year-old elementary school teacher*
Session Goal: General wellness support

Initial Observation (Visual & Tactile):
Upon intake, Mary presented no specific health concerns beyond general fatigue. However, during the foot scan, the pads directly beneath all ten toes (particularly in the lung and sinus reflex zones) felt **puffy**, slightly **spongy**, and **cooler than the surrounding tissue**. There was no evident discoloration, but the area lacked tone and firmness, giving it a "water-retaining" sensation under the practitioner's thumbs. These signs often correlate with sinus congestion, lymphatic stagnation, or unresolved respiratory tension.

Practitioner Technique Used:
Standard reflexology protocol was applied with a gentle return to the upper pads of the foot multiple times throughout the session. Pressure was modulated based on mild tenderness. The practitioner used alternating thumb-walking motions combined with light lymphatic drainage techniques toward the dorsal side.

Client Feedback During Session:
When asked if she felt anything during stimulation of the sinus/lung zone, Mary described a "weird sensitivity" but dismissed it as nothing significant. No acute pain or notable reaction occurred—just a dull, bloated tenderness.

Practitioner Notes:
The disconnect between the physical foot signs and the client's verbal response warranted a gentle probe. Using non-leading language, the practitioner asked, "Have you noticed any patterns with congestion or fatigue that you've been ignoring?" This allowed Mary to reflect rather than feel questioned.

Revealed Insight:
Mary admitted she had been **waking up congested for several months**, chalking it up to seasonal allergies. She hadn't connected it to her chronic fatigue and hadn't brought it up to her physician yet.

Outcome:
Following a few more sessions focusing on respiratory reflexes and draining patterns, Mary was referred by her physician for a sinus scan. The results confirmed **chronic sinusitis**, which had likely gone undetected for a long time due to its low-grade, persistent nature.

Client Reflection (Session 4):
Mary shared that after reflexology "brought the pressure to the surface," she felt more empowered to speak with her doctor. She noticed her sleep improved slightly after each session and remarked, "It was like my feet knew before I did."

Practitioner Takeaway:

- **Visual and textural cues**—even in the absence of verbal complaints—can reveal underlying imbalances worth gently exploring.
- Puffy pads beneath the toes, especially when **cool and untoned**, are often tied to **upper respiratory stagnation** and may signal sinus, lymphatic, or low-grade lung strain.
- Use **open-ended, reflective questions** rather than suggestive language to invite client awareness without leading.
- Encourage clients to notice patterns between sessions (e.g., breathing, sleep, energy) to build connection between their body's messages and their lived experience.

Case 2: Hollow Heels and Emotional Loss

Client: *"David," a 58-year-old widower*
Session Goal: Support for fatigue, tension relief

Initial Observation (Visual & Tactile):
During the initial foot scan, the **inner heel** zone on the **left foot** presented with a notable **hollowed-out dip**, both in appearance and tactile depth. The tissue felt **cool, slightly dehydrated,** and lacked the usual resistance or density found in the right heel. The skin in this area also had a faint gray hue and a papery texture—often associated with stagnation or underactivity in the corresponding reproductive and urinary reflex zones.

Practitioner Technique Used:
Due to the hollowness and sensitivity, the practitioner used **light pulsing and slow thumb-walking** in the inner heel area, focusing on restoring warmth and circulation. Lymphatic flushing was gently incorporated around the ankle zone to support elimination.

Client Feedback During Session:
David said he felt "a strange emptiness" when pressure was applied to the left heel and described the sensation as "ghost-like." He seemed emotionally distant but did not elaborate further during the session.

Practitioner Notes:
The stark contrast between the left and right heel, along with the somatic impression of "absence," prompted the practitioner to **ask neutrally**:

"Sometimes the feet reflect when the body has been through a loss or shift—has there been any major change in the past year?"

This opened the door without imposing a diagnosis or emotional prompt.

Revealed Insight:
David quietly shared that he had **lost his wife a year earlier** and had been in a prolonged state of emotional shutdown. After a pause, he added that he had undergone a **prostate procedure** six months prior but hadn't thought it relevant to mention. He explained that his fatigue had deepened since the procedure and that his sense of "being disconnected" was hard to shake.

Outcome (After Session 3):
David began attending sessions weekly and slowly reported **improved sleep, slight emotional release (tearfulness after sessions), and less pelvic tension.** He said,

"I didn't think my feet would remember more than I did. But I guess they didn't forget."

His left heel gradually regained warmth and tone over the next month of treatment, and he began participating in grief counseling through a local support group.

Practitioner Takeaway:

- **Hollow or sunken areas**, especially when accompanied by **coolness and graying**, may reflect **energetic depletion**, trauma, organ removal, or long-term suppression.
- The **left foot**, often tied to emotional or feminine energy, may store grief and relational wounding—especially in cases of spousal or maternal loss.
- Tactile indicators like **texture loss** and **temperature drop** in reflex zones can signal more than physical issues—they may reflect a **disconnection from self** or a **refusal to process**.

- Asking **neutral, non-leading questions** can gently bring awareness to the client without intruding.
- Emotional loss often imprints first in the **reproductive, kidney, adrenal, and heel reflexes**—zones tied to survival, grounding, and attachment.

Case 3: Calluses on the Fifth Toe and Smoking History

Client: *"Leanne," a 36-year-old retail manager*
Session Goal: General wellness and stress relief

Initial Observation (Visual & Tactile):
The client presented with **dense, yellowish calluses beneath both fifth toes**, extending slightly toward the lateral edge of the foot. The texture was thick, rough, and required more pressure to access the underlying reflex. This area corresponds to the **lung zone** in reflexology—commonly associated with respiratory health, breath capacity, and emotional expression.

Practitioner Technique Used:
Given the callus density, the practitioner softened the area using a warm compress and light oil, followed by **gentle circular friction** and **thumb pressure**. Care was taken not to overwork the area, as thick calluses may mask tenderness beneath the surface.

Client Response During Session:
Leanne reported a **dull ache** during pressure on the reflex point, saying it "felt like something was stuck there." When asked if she'd ever had lung-related issues or respiratory strain, she initially said no—but added that she used to smoke.

Revealed Insight:
On further conversation, Leanne shared she had **smoked for 15 years**, starting in her teens and quitting three years prior. She noted she had **never had any severe lung problems**, but had often experienced tightness in her chest during high-stress years in her twenties.

Her response to the reflex connection was both surprised and validating.

"I didn't know this spot was related to the lungs... it kind of feels like my body's way of showing what it's been through."

Practitioner Notes:
The **fifth toe/lung reflex callus** is a **frequent marker** among past or present smokers, individuals exposed to air pollutants, and those who habitually hold their breath under stress. The body may retain this memory in the reflex zone long after the behavior ends—like a **cellular scar or imprint**.

Outcome (After Session 2):
By the second session, the client noted that she was **more aware of her breathing patterns**, especially when stressed. She began practicing **breathwork exercises** between sessions. The calluses softened over time with consistent hydration, exfoliation, and reflex work, and Leanne reported **feeling "clearer" in both breath and mood**.

Practitioner Takeaway:

- **Calluses are not just physical foot problems—they are energetic reminders of wear, protection, or repetitive strain**.
- The **lung reflex** beneath the fifth toe can signal both physical issues (asthma, bronchitis, smoking history) and **emotional repression**, especially related to grief or "not being able to breathe in life."
- Clients who have **"moved on" from a habit like smoking** may still carry the **somatic echo** of that time, and recognizing it in the feet can open a healing dialogue.
- Use **supportive language** to affirm the body's intelligence, rather than framing signs as "damage."
- Complementary techniques like **breath awareness, salt soaks, and fascia release** can aid the transition to healthier respiratory patterns.

Case 4: Goosebump Texture and Undiagnosed Skin Issue

Client: *"Arjun," a 48-year-old engineer*
Session Goal: Support for ongoing digestive discomfort and low energy

Initial Observation (Visual & Tactile):
Upon palpating the **left arch**—corresponding to the **liver, small intestine, and digestive reflex zones**—the practitioner noted a **distinct goosebump-like texture**. The sensation was **raised, dry, and slightly coarse**, resembling fine bumps beneath the skin. Despite using warmth, this texture **persisted without softening**, which is atypical for standard skin dehydration or chills.

Practitioner Technique Used:
The area was gently worked using **circular fingertip brushing** and **cross-fiber friction**, alternating with warming compresses. The reflex remained **texturally resistant**, prompting deeper inquiry.

Client Report During Session:
Arjun shared he'd been experiencing **ongoing digestive irregularity**, bloating, and occasional nausea after meals. When asked about **skin concerns**, he hesitated, then mentioned a **mild, generalized itching** that "comes and goes" but hadn't caused visible rash or lesions. He had not yet sought medical advice.

Insight & Practitioner Follow-Up:
The persistent raised texture in the arch, **despite heat or hydration**, stood out as a **non-responsive tactile indicator**, often suggestive of **internal inflammation or immune response**. The practitioner gently encouraged Arjun to consult a dermatologist—not in alarm, but as a **preventive measure** to rule out skin hypersensitivity or systemic triggers.

"Reflexology can't diagnose, but sometimes the body whispers in ways that are worth listening to."

Outcome:
Two weeks later, Arjun returned and reported that his dermatologist had diagnosed him with a **mild autoimmune skin disorder** in its early stages (likely **lichen planus or eczema-form dermatitis**). The condition had not yet appeared on the skin's surface but was beginning to affect nerve endings and tissues beneath.

The reflexology session became the **first indicator** that something beneath the surface was at play.

Client Quote:

"I didn't expect my foot to tell me something before a doctor did."

Practitioner Takeaway:

- A **goosebump texture** that doesn't respond to warmth or hydration may suggest **early immune activity**, nervous system irritability, or **inflammatory skin disorders**.
- The **arch zone** corresponds to liver, intestines, and energy metabolism—frequent contributors to **autoimmune flare-ups** and **digestive-skin connections**.
- Reflexology is not diagnostic but can serve as an **early alert system**. Practitioners should **document, observe, and gently suggest appropriate referrals**.
- This case highlights the importance of **trusting your hands**—unusual or persistent textures are often worth exploring further.
- **Complementary support**: Incorporate **lymphatic drainage reflex techniques**, skin-soothing essential oils

(like **chamomile or lavender**), and **digestive dietary awareness** in follow-up care.

.

Case 5: Redness in the Digestive Zone & Emotional Stress

Client: *"Sofia," a 29-year-old graduate student*
Session Goal: General wellness support during exam season

Initial Observation (Visual & Tactile):
The **arch area on both feet**, corresponding to the **digestive reflex zones** (stomach, pancreas, intestines), appeared **bright red and warm to the touch**. The reflexes were slightly **spongy**, and pressure in these zones elicited a quick withdrawal—suggesting **heightened sensitivity or reactivity**.

Practitioner Technique Used:
Applied **gentle alternating pressure**, followed by **solar plexus and adrenal reflex work** to calm the nervous system. Techniques were modified to avoid overstimulation due to heat and tenderness in the area.

Client Report During Session:
When asked about digestive health, Sofia stated everything was "fine," although she admitted to being "just a bit stressed." No formal complaints were given initially.

Subtle Clues:

- Heat and coloration pointed toward **sympathetic nervous system dominance**
- Reactivity indicated the **gut-brain axis** may be under strain

- The symmetrical presence on both feet suggested **systemic emotional or hormonal stress,** rather than a localized physical dysfunction

Follow-Up Conversation:
At the close of the session, Sofia confided that she had been experiencing **daily stomach cramping,** tension headaches, and **difficulty sleeping**. These symptoms had intensified under the weight of her graduate workload, but she hadn't spoken to anyone, believing her stress wasn't "serious enough."

Outcome:
Within two weeks and after another reflexology session, Sofia reported feeling calmer and more in control. She decided to meet with a university counselor and described the reflexology as a **"turning point that made me stop ignoring the signs."**

"I thought I was just tired. I didn't realize how much my body was holding."

Practitioner Takeaway:

- **Redness + heat** in the **arch (digestive zone)** can point to **nervous system overload**, not just dietary causes. This may be especially true in high-functioning individuals minimizing their stress.
- **Emotional stress** often manifests physically in the **gut reflexes,** even when verbal reports seem unrelated.
- Reflexology offers an opportunity for **safe emotional release** and can create space for clients to **self-disclose without pressure**.
- Be mindful not to "push" emotionally—use **neutral language and gentle presence** to invite deeper awareness.

Complementary Support Suggestions:

- Recommend **breathing practices** or **vagal nerve stimulation** through footwork and guided relaxation
- Introduce **digestive-calming herbs** such as chamomile or lemon balm
- Encourage hydration and simple grounding rituals (warm foot soaks, walking barefoot on grass)
- When appropriate, suggest counseling or emotional wellness resources

Why These Cases Matter

Each of these examples shows that the feet *remember*—even when the mind forgets, minimizes, or delays acknowledgement. The signs we see or feel are often the first whispers from the body, and through skilled, compassionate reflexology, we help bring those whispers into awareness.

While every body is different, the patterns are real—and they can be incredibly validating for both client and practitioner.

What Clients Have Confirmed About the Common Signs

Over decades of practice, I have recorded thousands of "Yes, that's me!" moments—times when a client's lived experience matched exactly what their feet were broadcasting. While no single sign is diagnostic, the **consistency of these confirmations** shows how remarkably accurate the language of the feet can be.

Foot Sign	Typical Client Confirmation	Representative Quote
Persistent Redness on balls of feet or toes	Recent flare-ups of **migraines, sinus infections, reflux, or panic episodes**	"I've had heartburn all week—how did you know it was active today?"
Puffiness / Swelling (arch, under toes, ankle)	**Allergies, asthma, sinusitis, menstrual cramps, IVF treatments**	"My sinuses have been so stuffed; that puffiness makes sense now."
Hollow Zones (inner heel, arch)	**Organ removal**, long-standing fatigue, post-surgical numbness	"Yes—I had my gallbladder out years ago and that area feels empty."
Bony Protrusions / Ridges (dorsal shoulder line, outer foot)	Past **fractures, frozen shoulder, scoliosis, desk-job posture**	"That's the exact shoulder I tore in college."

Foot Sign	Typical Client Confirmation	Representative Quote
Gritty / Sandy Texture (kidneys, colon)	Kidney stones, gout, constipation, IBS; detox reactions after sessions	"Right after you worked there I had to run to the bathroom—it was a release."
Calluses (big toe, fifth toe, heel)	Heart strain, smoking history, sciatic pain, emotional 'armor'	"I quit smoking five years ago—funny that the callus is still protecting that spot."
Temperature Imbalance (one foot cold, one hot)	Thyroid issues, adrenal fatigue, localized inflammation	"My right knee is inflamed—that's the side that felt hot."
Toe Deformities (hammer, Morton's, overlapping)	Neck tension, TMJ, dental work, perfectionism	"I've worn a night-guard for jaw clenching since I got braces."
White Glow Under Toenail	Concussion history, brain fog, hormone migraines	"I hit my head snowboarding last year—didn't think my toe would show that!"
Excess Sweating / Foot Odor	Hyper-stress, blood-sugar swings, liver overload, puberty/menopause	"I sweat through my shoes during exams—exactly when my anxiety spikes."

Foot Sign	Typical Client Confirmation	Representative Quote
Heel Calluses / Cracks	IBS, constipation, pelvic tension, root-chakra insecurity	"When my IBS flares, the cracks always split deeper."
Ankle Puffiness (inner/outer)	Sciatica, ovarian cysts, testicular pain, lymph stagnation	"My sciatic nerve has been killing me—no wonder that ankle is swollen."
Shoulder Ridge Tightness (dorsal foot)	Daily caretaker stress, desk work, feeling 'burdened'	"I literally feel like I carry everyone on my shoulders—now I see it on my feet."

Key Patterns Observed

1. **Timing:** Signs often **precede medical diagnosis**—clients return later saying, "The doctor just confirmed what you felt in my feet."
2. **Emotion–Body Link:** Physical confirmations almost always include an **emotional component** (grief with lung puffiness, control issues with hammer toes, etc.).
3. **Session-to-Session Shifts:** When a reflex area softens or warms over multiple visits, clients report parallel improvements—fewer migraines, lighter periods, calmer digestion.
4. **Surprise Factor:** The most common response after a match is amazement:

   "I never mentioned that—how could my feet know?"

Why These Confirmations Matter

- They **validate the client's intuition**: what they "feel" finds a physical echo, building body trust.
- They help us **tailor after-care**: confirming a sign allows for more precise referrals—be it a dentist for TMJ or a gastroenterologist for reflux.
- They demonstrate that reflexology is a **two-way conversation**: the body speaks; we listen; the client hears their own story told back through objective sensation.

How Signs Evolved Over Time with Treatment

One of the most fascinating aspects of reflexology—especially when practiced consistently and consciously—is **watching the body reveal its healing journey** over time. The feet don't just reflect imbalances or tension in a static way; they show change, progress, and integration. Signs that were once rigid, swollen, gritty, or inflamed often soften, shrink, or even disappear entirely as the body responds to care.

Common Patterns of Evolution Observed:

Gritty or Sandy Texture

- **Before:** Grit in the kidney, colon, or sinus reflexes usually indicated stagnation, poor elimination, or toxin buildup.
- **After 3–5 sessions:** The texture would often reduce noticeably, becoming smoother and more fluid to the touch.
- **Client feedback:** "My bloating is down," or "I've been going to the bathroom more regularly."

Redness and Puffiness

- **Before:** Puffiness and redness in the ball of the foot or around the toes typically showed inflammation, acute stress, or overactivity (e.g., digestive flare-ups, asthma, reflux).
- **Over time:** The swelling recedes, skin tone normalizes, and the area may even appear slightly sunken for a while before rebalancing.

- **Client feedback:** "My heartburn has stopped," or "I'm not waking up wheezing anymore."

Temperature Shifts

- **Before:** Cold areas (especially heels or outer ankles) pointed to adrenal fatigue, hypothyroidism, or chronic tension.
- **With repeated sessions:** Temperature becomes more even, and clients report warmer feet and hands, better sleep, and more energy.
- **Client feedback:** "I don't need socks in bed anymore," or "My hands don't go numb like before."

Calluses and Cracks

- **Before:** Heel calluses or big-toe roughness often revealed bowel issues, suppressed grief, or long-term coping mechanisms.
- **Over time:** Skin softened, cracks reduced, and the protective hardness dissolved when deeper healing took place.
- **Client feedback:** "My IBS calmed down," or "I finally cried after years of holding it in."

Rigid or Curled Toes

- **Before:** Curled, overlapping, or hammer toes correlated with spinal tension, emotional rigidity, or postural compensation.
- **Gradual change:** While structure may not fully reverse, clients often regain flexibility, circulation, and even experience pain relief.
- **Client feedback:** "It doesn't cramp like before," or "I can wiggle that toe now."

White Glow Under Toenails

- **Before:** A pale, almost fluorescent glow beneath the nails signified brain overload—often seen in those recovering from concussion, trauma, or high cortisol states.
- **With regulation:** The glow fades, toenail beds pinken, and clients report improved focus, less anxiety, or decreased migraines.
- **Client feedback:** "I'm not as foggy," or "I've been sleeping better than I have in years."

The Bigger Picture

These changes do **not happen in isolation**. They evolve in tandem with:

- **Lifestyle changes** clients make (better hydration, food choices, stress reduction)
- **Other therapies** they are receiving (chiropractic, acupuncture, counseling)
- **Energetic shifts** that allow emotional release and integration

Tracking these changes over time helps practitioners:

- Build **confidence** in what they observe
- Deepen **rapport** with clients by celebrating wins together
- Refine treatment plans by knowing when to support, pause, or refer out

In reflexology, healing is not about forcing change—it's about creating the conditions where the body begins to speak differently.

How to Ask for Feedback Without Leading the Client

As reflexologists, we rely on **observation**, **experience**, and **client feedback** to deepen our understanding of what's happening in the body. However, the way we phrase our questions matters just as much as what we feel beneath our hands.

It is important not to **suggest**, **assume**, or **implant** an idea into the client's mind. Doing so not only compromises their response—it can create fear, confusion, or false memories.

Instead, aim to ask **open-ended, curiosity-based questions** that empower clients to reflect and share their experience.

Use Neutral, Open-Ended Language:

These phrases invite feedback without suggesting a diagnosis or condition.

- "I noticed some tenderness here—have you felt anything unusual in that part of your body lately?"
- "This area feels different today. Have you experienced any recent changes or stress?"
- "Is there anything you're aware of in terms of digestion (or breathing, or sleep) right now?"
- "This reflex feels slightly more reactive than usual. Does that resonate with how you've been feeling?"
- "That spot was a little puffy—have you felt congested or bloated recently?"

Avoid Leading or Suggestive Language:

These types of phrases can make the client feel alarmed, judged, or misinformed.

- "Do you have liver disease?"
- "This feels like cancer."
- "Your gallbladder might be failing."
- "This definitely means you have a hormone problem."
- "I think your uterus was removed—am I right?"

Tone Matters

Even a neutral question can feel intrusive if asked with intensity or urgency. The tone should always be:

- Calm
- Curious
- Supportive
- Respectful

Avoid trying to "be right." The goal is not to impress the client with your knowledge—it's to invite reflection and support their healing.

When to Simply Observe and Record

In some cases, you may notice a sign (like a hollow or callus) but choose not to bring it up—especially if:

- It's the client's first session
- They seem emotionally fragile or overly suggestible
- It does not impact your work in that moment

Instead, simply **record your observation** in your notes, revisit the area gently, and wait for the right moment to ask—perhaps in a future session when more trust is built.

Sample Follow-Up Prompts

Use these prompts to invite dialogue *after* the session:

- "How did that area feel to you today?"
- "Was there a part of the session that stood out?"
- "Have you noticed any shifts in your body after today's session?"
- "Would you like to explore more about that tenderness next time?"

Your words have power. Use them wisely. When you hold space for discovery—not prediction—you build trust, credibility, and deeper healing outcomes.

Chapter 11: Complementary Therapies & Recommendations

When and How to Refer

Integrating Reflexology with a Holistic Wellness Team

As powerful as reflexology is, it is most effective **as part of a larger wellness ecosystem**. Knowing when to refer your client to another professional is not just ethical—it's a sign of maturity and confidence as a practitioner. True healing is collaborative.

When to Refer: Recognizing the Signs

Clients may benefit from complementary therapies when:

- **Progress plateaus:** If symptoms persist after several sessions with no change.
- **Deeper layers surface:** Emotional releases, trauma responses, or intense dreams indicate a need for counseling or emotional support.

- **You feel out of scope:** If symptoms suggest structural misalignment, hormonal issues, unresolved injury, or systemic illness.
- **You notice physical limitations:** Such as rigid posture, visible scoliosis, jaw clenching, or nerve pain that may require chiropractic or physio support.

Who to Refer To — and Why

Massage Therapy

- **Best for:** Muscular tension, fascia restrictions, lymph drainage, stress relief.
- **Example:** When you feel hard or unresponsive muscle bands in the calves or heel zone.

Chiropractic

- **Best for:** Skeletal misalignments, nerve impingements, postural imbalances.
- **Example:** If the spine reflex feels painful or distorted, or toes indicate neck and jaw tension.

Acupuncture or Traditional Chinese Medicine (TCM)

- **Best for:** Energy blockages, organ imbalances, reproductive health, pain relief.
- **Example:** Puffy arches or energy depletion that don't shift with reflexology alone.

Counseling or Somatic Therapy

- **Best for:** Emotional trauma, unresolved grief, anxiety, or behavioral patterns affecting physical health.
- **Example:** When feet show consistent rigidity, disconnection, or glow under nails—paired with emotional disclosures.

Nutritionist or Holistic Health Coach

- **Best for:** Digestive issues, inflammation, hormonal imbalances, fatigue.
- **Example:** Puffy arches, gritty textures, or recurring inflammation near digestive reflex zones.

Naturopathic Doctor or Functional Medicine Practitioner

- **Best for:** Underlying chronic health issues, hormonal or metabolic concerns.
- **Example:** When adrenal reflexes feel depleted, or thyroid/circulation signs present chronically.

How to Refer with Grace and Confidence

Referrals should never imply that reflexology failed. Instead, frame them as an act of **whole-person care**:

- "I'm noticing something in the [specific reflex] area that may benefit from another layer of support."
- "Have you ever considered working with a [type of practitioner]? I think it could really complement what we're doing here."
- "This feels like a pattern that might go deeper than reflexology alone can shift. A professional in [field] may help you go further."

Documentation and Follow-Up

- **Record** what signs led to your referral suggestion (e.g., texture, pain, temperature).
- **Ask for permission** to check in after they've seen another provider.
- **Never diagnose** or contradict another healthcare provider's opinion.

Being a skilled reflexologist doesn't mean doing everything—it means knowing how to integrate your wisdom with the right support at the right time.

When reflexology becomes a **gateway to deeper healing**, you become more than a practitioner—you become a guide.

Nutrition and Hydration for Specific Zones & Signs

Supporting the Body from the Inside Out Based on Reflex Feedback

Reflexology doesn't diagnose—but it can reveal imbalances that point toward areas needing extra support. When certain textures, temperatures, or sensations arise in the feet, they often reflect the body's internal state. Through careful observation, practitioners can suggest supportive self-care tools—particularly through diet and hydration—without overstepping professional boundaries.

Digestive Zones (Arch, Heels, Inner Foot)

Common Signs:

- Gritty texture
- Puffiness
- Hollow or sunken areas

Supportive Nutrition:

- **Hydration:** Increase clean water intake, especially first thing in the morning. Add lemon or apple cider vinegar to stimulate digestion.
- **Bitter foods:** Arugula, dandelion greens, and artichokes support bile flow and liver detox.
- **Fermented foods:** Sauerkraut, kimchi, or kefir help nourish the gut microbiome.
- **Fiber:** Ground flaxseed, chia seeds, and leafy greens improve colon movement.

- **Avoid:** Excess sugar, processed carbs, or known sensitivities (e.g., dairy, gluten).

Heart and Lung Zones (Ball of Foot, Under Toes)

Common Signs:

- Puffiness or redness
- Stress or tension patterns
- Shallow or ridged skin texture

Supportive Nutrition:

- **Healthy fats:** Omega-3s from flaxseed oil, walnuts, and fish support cardiovascular and nervous system health.
- **Magnesium-rich foods:** Pumpkin seeds, almonds, and spinach help regulate stress and muscle tension.
- **Deep red/purple foods:** Beets, berries, and red cabbage support heart health and circulation.
- **Breath-supportive herbs:** Mullein, thyme, or peppermint teas can soothe lung reflexes.

Adrenal and Kidney Zones (Mid Arch, Medial Foot)

Common Signs:

- Puffiness, tenderness, or lack of resilience
- Hollow texture or temperature imbalance

Supportive Nutrition:

- **Sea salt or mineral-rich salts** (e.g., Celtic, Himalayan) to support electrolyte balance.
- **Adaptogens:** Ashwagandha, rhodiola, or licorice root (under guidance) help balance stress.
- **Vitamin C-rich foods:** Bell peppers, oranges, and kiwi bolster adrenal function.

- **Hydration:** Sufficient water—especially when under stress—is essential for adrenal and kidney function.

Brain and Nervous System Zones (Toes, Spine Zones)

Common Signs:

- White glow under nails
- Rigid or curled toes
- Tingling or numbness

Supportive Nutrition:

- **Essential fatty acids:** Avocados, wild-caught fish, flaxseed
- **B vitamins:** Eggs, whole grains, nutritional yeast (support nervous system repair)
- **Dark chocolate and green tea:** Moderate amounts support blood flow to the brain and mood elevation
- **Reduce stimulants:** Especially if signs of burnout or nerve irritation are present

Reproductive and Hormonal Zones (Heel, Ankle, Outer Foot)

Common Signs:

- Puffy or swollen tissue
- Dryness or calluses
- Tenderness around ovary/testicle reflex

Supportive Nutrition:

- **Hormone-balancing seeds:** Pumpkin/flax (follicular phase), sesame/sunflower (luteal phase)
- **Phytoestrogens:** Flaxseed, miso, legumes (especially helpful during perimenopause)

- **Cruciferous veggies:** Broccoli, cauliflower, and Brussels sprouts support estrogen detox
- **Water with electrolytes:** Supports pelvic circulation and tissue resilience

Hydration Tips for All Zones

- **Warm water sips throughout the day** support lymph flow better than large infrequent amounts.
- **Infused waters** (cucumber, mint, citrus) can encourage consistent intake.
- **Avoid excessive diuretics** (coffee, alcohol) if dry/cracked feet or cold zones are frequent.
- Encourage clients to view hydration as a healing tool—not just a habit.

Important Note: Rather than prescribing diets, you can say: "I've noticed this reflex area is puffy or gritty—sometimes that shows up when the body's working hard in that system. You might explore foods that support digestion/adrenals/etc., or chat with a nutritionist."

By connecting reflex signs with internal nourishment, you empower your clients to partner with their body—gently and intuitively.

Herbal Support, Essential Oils & Energy Clearing

Subtle Tools to Enhance Reflexology Insights

Reflexology reveals imbalances through texture, sensitivity, and energetic density—long before a medical diagnosis may appear. Once these signs are observed, gentle complementary tools like herbs, essential oils, and energetic clearing can help restore harmony across body, mind, and spirit.

Herbal Support by Zone or Symptom

1. Digestive Zones (Arch, Heels):

- **Peppermint** – Calms digestive spasms and tension.
- **Chamomile** – Soothes stomach and emotional stress.
- **Dandelion root** – Gently stimulates liver and bile flow.
- **Ginger** – Warming and improves gut motility.

Use teas or tinctures; best under guidance if client is on medication.

2. Adrenal & Kidney (Medial arch):

- **Nettle leaf** – Mineral-rich; nourishes adrenal fatigue.
- **Licorice root** – Supports adrenal function (avoid with high BP).
- **Ashwagandha** – Adaptogenic support for long-term stress.

3. Lung & Heart (Ball of foot):

- **Mullein** – Softens and clears lung congestion.
- **Hawthorn berry** – Tones and strengthens the heart.
- **Motherwort** – Calms anxiety-related heart flutter.

4. Reproductive (Heel, Ankle):

- **Vitex (Chasteberry)** – Supports hormonal regulation in women.
- **Red raspberry leaf** – Tones uterus and menstrual system.
- **Maca root** – Balances energy, stamina, and libido in both sexes.

Essential Oils for Reflex Zones

Apply "**diluted**" oils to corresponding foot zones, or use aromatically:

Reflex Zone	Suggested Oils	Benefits
Solar Plexus / Adrenals	Frankincense, Bergamot, Lavender	Calming and centering
Lungs	Eucalyptus, Tea Tree, Ravintsara	Clear congestion, purify breath
Liver	Lemon, Rosemary, Geranium	Detox support and energetic release
Colon/Digestion	Ginger, Fennel, Peppermint	Motility and inflammation support
Reproductive	Clary Sage, Rose, Ylang Ylang	Hormonal balance and comfort

Always use carrier oils. Avoid applying to broken or inflamed skin.

Energy Clearing Practices

Energy often becomes "stuck" in the feet—especially from trauma, unexpressed emotion, or overthinking. Consider adding:

1. Auric Sweeps

- Lightly hover your hands above the feet to sweep dense energy away. Visualize clearing fog or static.

2. Crystal Placement

- Use grounding stones (e.g., hematite, black tourmaline) at heels or beneath treatment table.
- Use calming stones (e.g., amethyst, selenite) near toes or head.

3. Reiki or Intentional Energy Channeling

- Gently channel energy into the feet after your reflexology sequence.
- Focus on bringing light and neutrality into hot, cold, or dense-feeling areas.

4. Sound Vibration

- Use tuning forks (especially weighted) around ankle zones or heel to reset nervous system.
- Crystal bowls with grounding tones (C for root, G for throat) can help release emotional holding.

Practitioner Tip:

When suggesting herbs or oils, you might say:
"In this reflex area, I'm noticing signs that often relate to
_____."

"Some people find that _____ (herb/oil)

helps them feel more balanced there. Let me know if you'd like
to explore that further or speak with an herbalist."

These subtle supports work beautifully alongside reflexology—
not to treat symptoms, but to support the body's natural wisdom
and energetic flow.

Journaling Prompts for Client Self-Awareness

Deepening the Healing Journey Beyond the Reflexology Session

Encouraging your clients to reflect on their experiences helps bridge body awareness with emotional insight. Journaling can reveal patterns, foster empowerment, and increase the effectiveness of reflexology by inviting the client into active participation in their healing.

Below are suggested journaling prompts organized by theme or concern. You may print or share them in follow-up materials or self-care programs.

General Body Awareness

- "What sensations stood out to me during today's session? Where did I feel tension, discomfort, or relief?"
- "If my feet could speak, what would they be trying to tell me?"
- "How have I felt physically this week—energized, drained, tight, or loose?"
- "Which parts of my body feel supported? Which feel ignored or overworked?"

Mental & Emotional Insight

- "Did anything emotional arise during or after my reflexology session?"
- "Are there thoughts I'm avoiding or looping through repeatedly?"

- "Where in my body do I carry emotional stress?"
- "What am I ready to let go of that no longer serves me?"

Left vs. Right Foot (Emotional vs. Physical)

- "What did I notice differently between my left and right foot?"
- "How might the issues on my left foot reflect emotional patterns or relationship stress?"
- "How might the issues on my right foot relate to daily habits or responsibilities?"

Lifestyle & Routine Check-In

- "How are my sleep, nutrition, and hydration patterns this week?"
- "What might my feet be revealing about my daily choices?"
- "Is there something in my life I'm 'standing on' or 'standing up for'—or not?"

Intuitive Reflection

- "When did I last feel truly grounded and connected to myself?"
- "What color, image, or word do I associate with the area that felt tender or blocked?"
- "What would my inner healer suggest I do for support right now?"

After a Series of Sessions

- "What has shifted for me physically, mentally, or emotionally since beginning reflexology?"
- "Which patterns keep reappearing, and what might they be teaching me?"
- "How do I feel now compared to my first session?"

Practitioner Tip: Encourage clients to journal right after their session, while sensations and insights are fresh. You can even give them a small notepad or email a printable prompt sheet. Journaling isn't just for writers—it's a dialogue with the self, and the feet are simply part of the language.

Practitioner Reflection Pages

For Personal Insight, Growth, and Better Client Outcomes

Including practitioner reflection pages in your notes or post-session journaling can elevate your reflexology practice. These pages serve as a space to deepen your clinical intuition, track patterns over time, refine your technique, and connect energetically and emotionally to your work.

Below are structured sections and sample prompts for use after each session—or for end-of-week reflection.

Session Overview

- **Client Name:**
- **Date:**
- **Focus Areas (client request or observed):**
- **Reflex Zones Noted (tension, texture, temp, etc.):**
- **Client Feedback During Session (verbal or non-verbal):**
- **Energy Flow Observations:**
- **Post-session impressions or themes:**

Patterns & Progress Tracking

- **What recurring signs or imbalances are showing up across sessions?**
- **Is there improvement in previously stagnant or inflamed zones?**

- Are the client's symptoms aligning with what I'm observing in their feet?
- How has the texture, tone, or temperature of the feet shifted over time?

Energetic & Emotional Awareness

- Was there an emotional or energetic shift during the session?
- How did *I* feel while working on the client? (energized, drained, centered, distracted?)
- Were any emotions mirrored or triggered in me that I need to process or clear?
- Is there something intuitive I sensed but didn't voice—should I revisit it next time?

Clinical or Technique Notes

- What techniques were most effective today? (e.g., thumb-walking, holds, energy sweep)
- Any tools used? (e.g., essential oils, tuning forks, crystals)
- Was my pressure or pacing aligned with the client's needs?
- What might I do differently next time to improve flow or outcome?

Personal Development Check-In

- What did this session teach me—as a practitioner or person?
- What themes are showing up in multiple clients (and myself) lately?
- What self-care or grounding do I need after today's sessions?
- Is there a training, resource, or modality I feel called to explore further?

Optional End-of-Week Reflections:

- Which sessions stood out to me most this week—and why?
- Am I practicing enough self-care to remain present and effective?
- What growth or improvement have I noticed in myself or my clients recently?

Closing Note:

These reflection pages aren't just for documentation—they're for energetic hygiene, confidence building, and developing your intuitive reflexology wisdom. The more you reflect, the more fluent you become in the language the feet are trying to speak.

APPENDIXS

Foot Charts

Bottom of The Feet Plantar View

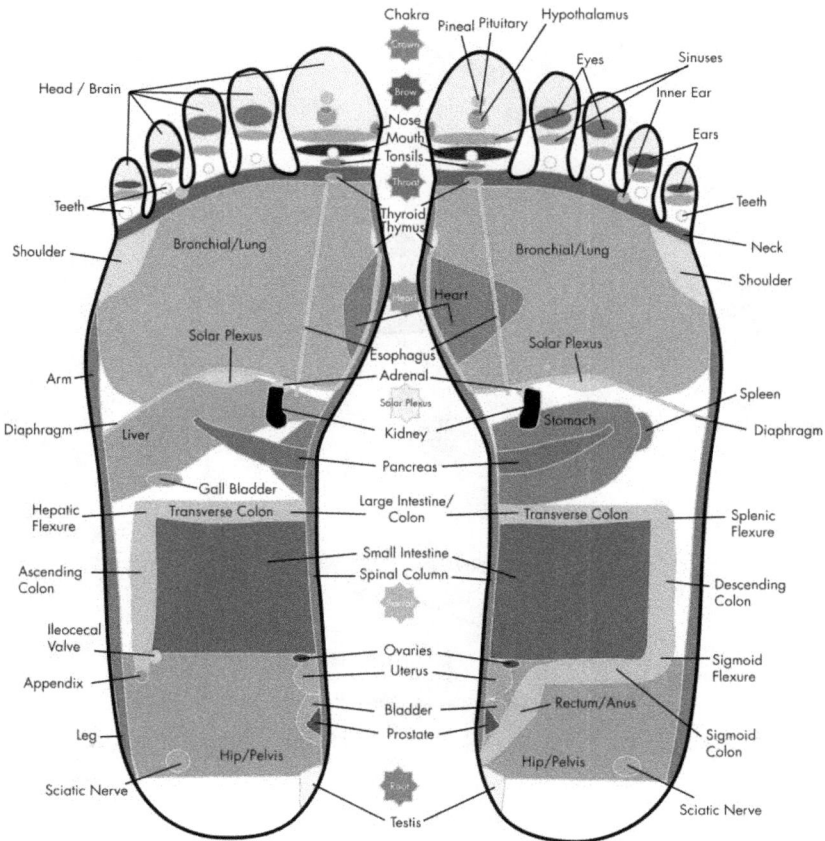

Chakra · Pineal · Pituitary · Hypothalamus
Crown
Eyes · Sinuses
Head / Brain
Brow
Inner Ear
Nose
Mouth · Ears
Tonsils
Throat
Teeth · Teeth
Thyroid/Thymus
Shoulder · Bronchial/Lung · Bronchial/Lung · Neck
Heart · Heart · Shoulder
Solar Plexus · Solar Plexus
Arm · Esophagus · Adrenal · Spleen
Solar Plexus
Diaphragm · Liver · Stomach · Diaphragm
Kidney
Pancreas
Gall Bladder · Large Intestine/Colon
Hepatic Flexure · Transverse Colon · Transverse Colon · Splenic Flexure
Small Intestine
Ascending Colon · Spinal Column · Descending Colon
Ileocecal Valve · Ovaries · Sigmoid Flexure
Uterus
Appendix · Bladder · Rectum/Anus
Leg · Prostate · Sigmoid Colon
Hip/Pelvis · Hip/Pelvis
Sciatic Nerve · Root · Sciatic Nerve
Testis

Dorsal / Back View

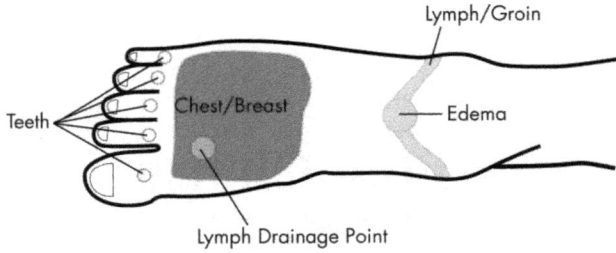

Lateral / Outside View

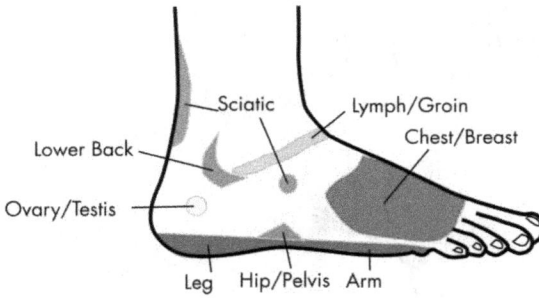

Medial / Inside View

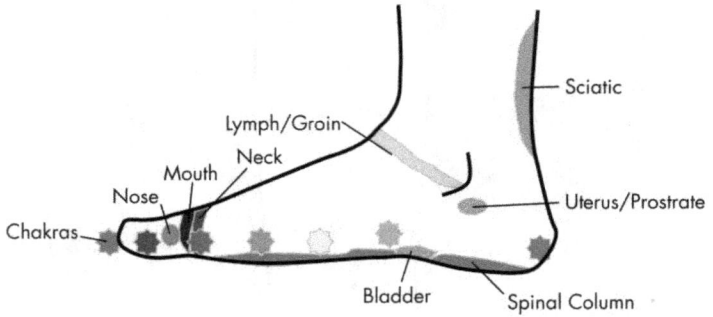

Hand Charts

Right Hand & Left Hand (Palmar View)

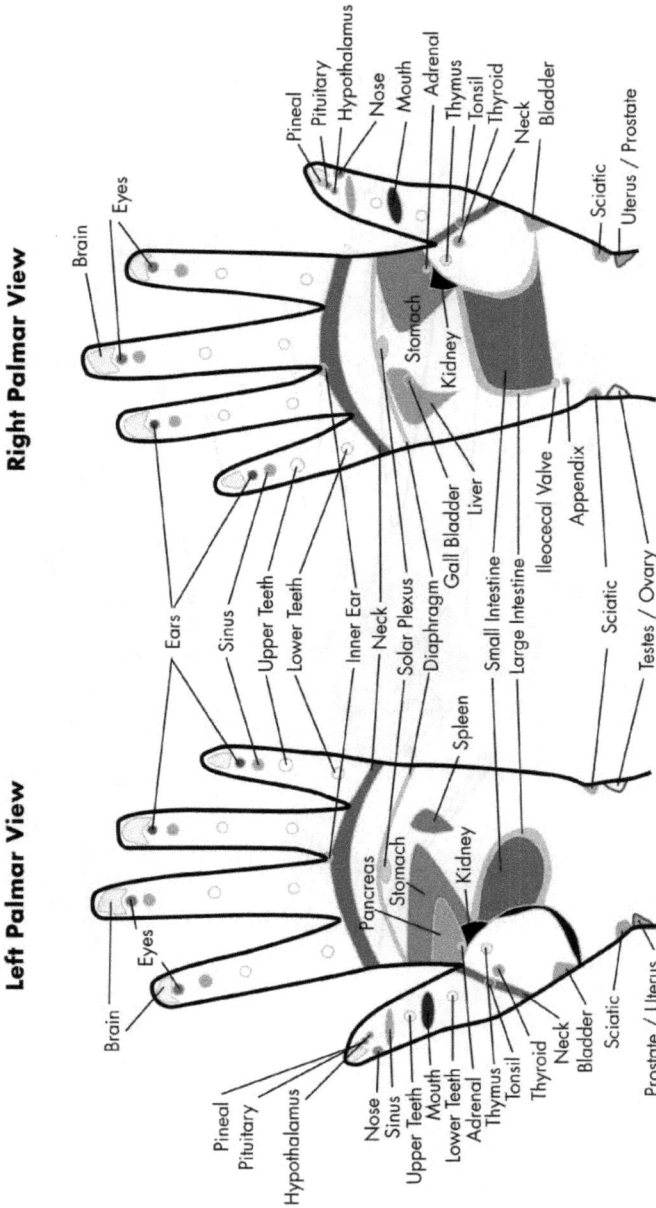

Right Palmar View

Pineal
Pituitary
Hypothalamus
Nose
Mouth
Adrenal
Thymus
Tonsil
Thyroid
Neck
Bladder
Sciatic
Uterus / Prostate
Eyes
Brain
Stomach
Kidney

Left Palmar View

Ears
Sinus
Upper Teeth
Lower Teeth
Inner Ear
Neck
Solar Plexus
Diaphragm
Gall Bladder
Liver
Small Intestine
Large Intestine
Ileocecal Valve
Appendix
Sciatic
Testes / Ovary
Spleen
Kidney
Pancreas
Stomach
Eyes
Brain
Pineal
Pituitary
Hypothalamus
Nose
Sinus
Upper Teeth
Mouth
Lower Teeth
Adrenal
Thymus
Tonsil
Thyroid
Neck
Bladder
Sciatic
Prostate / Uterus

Right Hand (Dorsal View)

The left hand is identical to the right on the back.

Dorsal / Back View

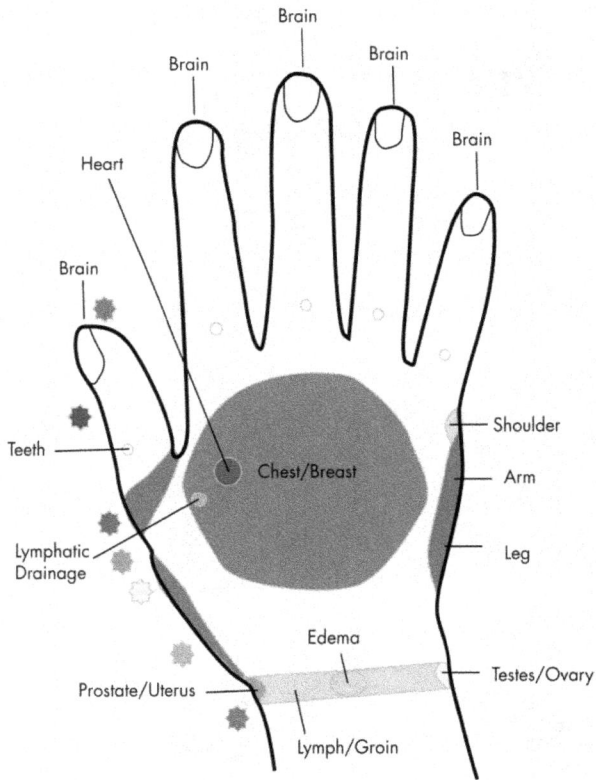

Zones

Vertical Zones

Vertical zones run through the length of the feet, legs, hands, arms, and body from front to back. There is a total of ten zones covering the whole body, with five zones on each side of the median line.

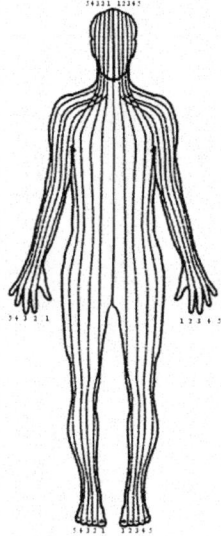

Dorsal View

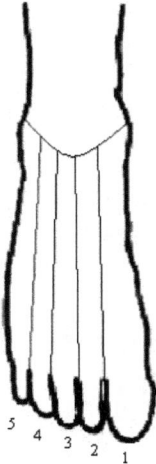

The Big Toe and Foot

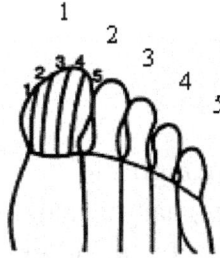

Lateral View

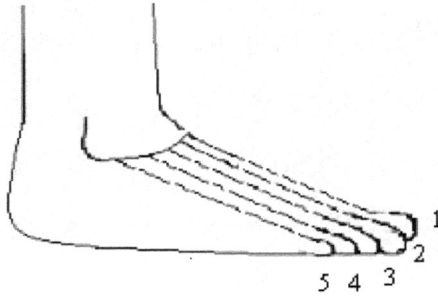

Horizontal Zones

Horizontal zones run from one side of
the foot to the other. Their borders may
not be perfectly straight;
however, they are most
useful for identifying the
location of reflexes.

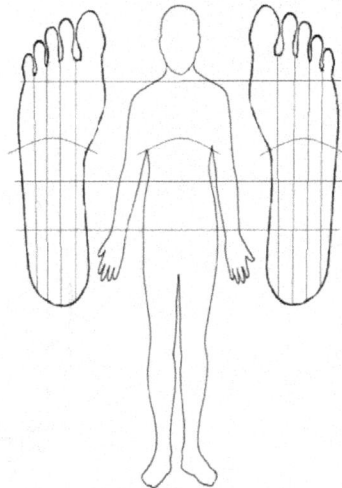

Reflexology Terms

These Reflexology terms are used in the following pages. Please refer to them throughout this course.

Butterfly Stretch: Similar to the Dorsal and Plantar Stretch; Stretching of the sole and the dorsal aspect using the fingers

Calcaneus: The heel bone

Carpals: The bones that form the wrist

Circumduction: Rotation of the foot

Compress: To press together

Cross over: Crossing from one side to the other

Distal: A part of the arm, leg, hand, or feet furthest from the main trunk

Dorsal: Pertaining to the back of the body or the back of hands and feet

Flexion: Bending the foot backward and forwards

Friction: Moving one surface over another, rubbing a surface of the body

Hook: Applying pressure by bending the first thumb joint and exerting pressure inwards while pulling back over the place with the thumb

Knead: To massage as if working bread dough

Knuckle press: Applying pressure with the knuckle of the fore or middle finger to a specific reflex

Knuckle Roll: Rolling the knuckles on the sole of the foot

Lateral: Pertaining to the side furthest from the median line

Medial: Pertaining to the middle line of the body

Metacarpals: The bones that form the palm of the hand, connecting the carpals to the phalanges or fingers

Palmar: The palm of the hand

Plantar: The sole of the foot

Plantar Stretch: A stretch of the sole or plantar part of the foot upwards, usually with the fingers of both hands, while the dorsal aspect is pushed downward by the thumbs and heel of the hand

Proximal: Part of the arm, leg, hand, or foot that is closest to the main trunk

Side Friction: A rapid movement of the palms of the hands against the sides of the foot; the fingers are slightly cupped and relaxed.

Slide: To move gently across a surface without losing contact

Spinal Twist: A gentle rotation or twisting of the foot, along with the spinal reflex, using both hands

Support Hand: The hand the holds the foot steady; the non-working hand

Sweep: Lightly pass over an area of the body with both hands, while barely touching the skin

Tarsals: The seven bones that form the heel (talus, calcaneus, navicular, cuboid and three cuneiform bones)

Thumb Rub: A gentle rubbing motion by the thumbs horizontally across the sole of the foot

Thumb Walk: Bending and straightening the first joint of the thumb by which the thumb moves forward

Torque: To cause rotation or twisting

Traction: The act of exerting a pulling force

Twist: To cause to rotate; to distort out of
natural shape

Working Hand: The hand doing the thumb or finger
walking

Zoning: Lightly thumb walking the five zones
of the toes or the foot

What This Might Mean —
Quick Reference Table

Foot Sign or Texture	Possible Meaning	Suggested Support
Redness (localized)	Inflammation, acute stress, or organ overactivity in that zone	Anti-inflammatory diet, calming techniques, reflexology
Puffiness (spongy tissue)	Lymph stagnation, fluid retention, emotional congestion	Lymphatic drainage, hydration, journaling
Gritty/sandy texture	Uric/lactic acid buildup, colon/kidney overload	Digestive support, detox practices, reflex point focus
Hollow or sunken areas	Organ disconnect, surgery/removal, emotional depletion	Energy healing, nourishment, adrenal support
Thick callus (specific area)	Chronic stress, suppression, or protective barrier	Emotional release, physical therapy, soften over time
Cool or cold area	Circulatory weakness, thyroid or adrenal fatigue	Warm foot baths, herbal support, circulation-focused massage

Foot Sign or Texture	Possible Meaning	Suggested Support
Hot/warm area (localized)	Inflammation or possible infection	Cooling compress, medical referral if persistent
Dry, cracked heels or toes	Poor hydration, lack of grounding, mineral deficiency	Grounding practices, foot soaks, increase water intake
White glow under toenails	Brain or nervous system tension, past trauma	Energy clearing, craniosacral work, journaling
Curled/rigid toes	Emotional holding, neurological tension, past trauma	Reflexology, trauma release work, somatic therapies
Vertical line between toes	Often linked to reflux or upper digestive tension	Nutrition review, stress reduction, acupuncture
Darkened toenail beds or tips	Circulatory concerns, unresolved grief, sluggish system	Emotional work, herbal tonics, grounding exercises
Goosebump-like skin texture	Nervous system activation, autoimmune sensitivity	Nervous system resets, adaptogens, light touch therapy
Bony protrusions (non-injury)	Chronic tension, skeletal misalignment, lack of energetic flexibility	Chiropractic care, posture alignment, fascia release

Foot Sign or Texture	Possible Meaning	Suggested Support
Puffy ankle (medial/lateral)	Hormonal issues, reproductive stress, or sciatic involvement	Hormone support, reflexology, yoga/stretching

This table can be printed and added as a **laminated chart** in your treatment room or included in the appendix of your book for fast practitioner reference.

Self-Assessment Checklist

What Are Your Feet Telling You?

Take a few quiet moments to examine your feet. Use a mirror or ask someone to help if needed. Check off anything that applies and journal your observations for later comparison.

General Observations

- ☐ My feet often feel cold to the touch
- ☐ My feet are frequently warm or flushed
- ☐ One foot looks or feels different than the other
- ☐ My feet swell by the end of the day
- ☐ I notice odor even with regular hygiene

Skin & Texture

- ☐ I have dry or cracked skin on my heels or toes
- ☐ There are calluses on specific areas (note location)
- ☐ I feel gritty or sandy texture under the skin when massaging my feet
- ☐ My skin feels unusually thick or hard in places
- ☐ I have soft or puffy tissue in certain zones

Color & Temperature

- ☐ I see red, purple, or dark patches
- ☐ Certain areas appear pale or have a white glow
- ☐ My feet change color depending on time of day or activity
- ☐ My feet often feel numb, tingling, or "buzzing"

Toenails & Nail Beds

- ☐ My toenails are discolored or brittle
- ☐ There's a white glow under one or more nails
- ☐ I have a history of fungal issues
- ☐ The nails grow at uneven angles

Toes & Alignment

- ☐ I have curled, bent, or rigid toes (e.g., hammer toes)
- ☐ My toes overlap or are widely spaced
- ☐ One or more toes show visible swelling or redness
- ☐ I've had dental work or jaw issues (check dorsal toe tension)

Arches & Posture

- ☐ I have flat feet or very high arches
- ☐ My weight distribution feels uneven when I walk or stand
- ☐ My feet feel tired or sore even after short walks
- ☐ I wear orthotics or supportive footwear daily

Emotional & Energetic Cues

- ☐ My feet often feel "heavy," disconnected, or numb
- ☐ I experience tension or anxiety held in the feet
- ☐ I feel grounded and supported through my feet (positive)
- ☐ I've experienced trauma, and notice it shows up physically

What to Do With This Information:

- Review any patterns you checked off.
- Compare both feet—note symmetry or lack thereof.
- Journal how your feet feel before and after self-care or treatment.
- Bring your notes to a reflexology or holistic session for discussion.
- Remember: This is a tool for awareness, not diagnosis.

Client Intake Form Template

Client Name:

_____

Date: _____
Date of Birth: _____
Phone/Email:

_____

Referred By:

_____

Primary Concern/Reason for Visit:

_____

_____

Medical History (check all that apply):
☐ Heart issues   ☐ Digestive concerns   ☐ Diabetes
☐ Hormonal imbalance   ☐ Chronic stress   ☐
Anxiety/Depression
☐ Spinal/back problems ☐ Pregnancy   ☐
Circulatory issues
☐ Arthritis   ☐ Previous surgeries (list):

_____

Current Medications & Supplements:

_____

_____

Lifestyle Notes:

- Water Intake (cups/day): _____
- Sleep Quality (1–10): _____
- Energy Level (1–10): _____
- Exercise Routine:

  _____

- Any known allergies or sensitivities?

  _____

Consent & Disclaimer:

I understand that reflexology is not a substitute for medical care and that the practitioner does not diagnose or prescribe. I give consent for this session.

Signature: _____   **Date:**

_____

Reflexology Session Notes Template

Client Name: _____

Session Date: _____   **Session #:** _____

Observations (Before Session):

☐ Skin: __ Dry __ Oily __ Normal   ☐ Cracks/Calluses (location): _____

☐ Puffiness/Edema: __ Yes __ No   ☐ Temperature: __ Cold __ Warm __ Mixed

☐ Discoloration: __ Red __ Pale __ Blue/Purple __ Other:

_____

☐ Texture: __ Gritty __ Soft __ Firm __ Swollen __ Sensitive

Foot Shape/Arch:

__ Flat __ Normal __ High   Symmetry: __ Symmetrical __ Asymmetrical

Postural/Structural Notes:

_____

_____

Zones & Reflexes Noted as Tender/Imbalanced:
☐ Toes – (describe):

_____

☐ Ball of Foot –

_____

☐ Arch –

_____

☐ Heel –

_____

☐ Dorsal Foot –

_____

Emotional or Verbal Cues from Client:

_____

Session Focus:
☐ General Balancing   ☐ Specific Zone Support   ☐
Emotional Release
☐ Stress Relief   ☐ Pain Management   ☐ Other:

_____

Changes During Session:
☐ Temperature shift   ☐ Sweating   ☐ Tension release   ☐
Breath change
☐ Verbal feedback   ☐ Energy shift   ☐ Emotional response

Post-Session Observations & Recommendations:

_____

_____

Home Care Suggestions (if any):

☐ Hydration   ☐ Gentle self-massage   ☐ Journaling   ☐ Rest

☐ Nutrition Focus: _____

☐ Referral to: _____

Practitioner Notes & Reflections:

_____

_____

Practitioner Signature: _____

Date: _____

Practitioner's Ethical Checklist

☐ **Stay Within Scope of Practice**

- Never diagnose medical conditions.
- Never prescribe medications, supplements, or treatment plans.
- Always refer out when unsure or when signs raise concern.

☐ **Describe Reflexes, Not Organs**

- Say: "This reflex point is tender."
- Avoid: "You have a problem with your liver."

☐ **Use Non-Directive, Observational Language**

- Focus on what is felt, seen, or sensed.
- Invite clients to share their experiences.

☐ **Ask Permission Before Touch**

- Especially if working around sensitive areas (ankles, inner arch, reproductive reflexes).

☐ **Maintain Client Confidentiality**

- Keep all records secure and private.
- Anonymize any shared stories (even for training or books).

☐ Stay Curious, Not Predictive

- Avoid suggesting outcomes or creating fear.
- Focus on potential support and awareness.

☐ Practice Cultural Sensitivity and Inclusivity

- Be mindful of diverse health beliefs, gender identity, and trauma-informed care.

☐ Keep Records Neutrally

- Use objective wording (e.g., "Tender at medial arch reflex" rather than "Colon issues").

☐ Honor Client Autonomy

- Encourage them to make decisions in partnership with licensed professionals.
- Provide information, not direction.

☐ Commit to Continuing Education

- Stay updated on anatomy, energy medicine ethics, and trauma-informed care.

Suggested Language Guide

Situation	Instead of Saying...	Say This...
Reflex is tender	"You have liver issues."	"The liver reflex point feels tender—have you noticed any changes in digestion or energy lately?"
Skin tone unusual	"You look pale; your circulation must be bad."	"There's some paleness in this area—sometimes that can relate to circulation. Have you noticed cold feet or fatigue?"
Gritty area found	"You have toxin buildup."	"There's a grainy texture here, which often shows up when this zone needs support."
Emotional release	"You're holding trauma."	"Sometimes this area can store stress—do you feel like your body holds tension here?"
Suggesting next steps	"You need to do a detox."	"If you're open, a naturopath or nutritionist may offer support for what we're noticing here."

BIBLIOGRAPHY

Much of this information was created and copywritten

- **Ingham, Eunice D.** *Stories the Feet Can Tell Thru Reflexology.* St. Petersburg, FL: Ingham Publishing, 1938.
- **Ingham, Eunice D.** *Stories the Feet Have Told.* St. Petersburg, FL: Ingham Publishing, 1951.
- **Fitzgerald, William H.** *Zone Therapy; or Relieving Pain at Home.* New York: J.S. Ogilvie Publishing, 1917.
- **Riley, Dr. Joe Shelby.** *Zone Therapy Simplified.* Washington, D.C., 1919.
- **Bowers, Edwin F.** *To Stop That Toothache, Squeeze Your Toe!* (Magazine Article, 1915).
- **Tiran, Denise.** *Reflexology in Pregnancy and Childbirth.* Edinburgh: Churchill Livingstone, 2010.
- **Keet, Ann Gillanders.** *The Family Guide to Reflexology.* New York: Fireside, 1992.
- **Dougans, Inge.** *Reflexology: The 5 Elements and Their 12 Meridians – A Unique Approach.* London: Thorsons, 1996.
- **Seymour, Laura Norman.** *The Reflexology Handbook.* London: Piatkus Books, 1989.
- **Hall, Christine Issel.** *Reflexology: Art, Science and History.* Sacramento: New Frontier Publishing, 1990.
- **Shapiro, Shira.** *Reflexology: The Healing Art of Touch.* New York: Healing Arts Press, 1996.
- **McVicar, J.** *The Complete Illustrated Guide to Reflexology.* London: Element Books, 1997.
- **Wright, Barbara and Kevin Kunz.** *Hand and Foot Reflexology: A Self-Help Guide.* New York: Prentice Hall, 1983.

- **Bach, Edward.** *Heal Thyself.* London: CW Daniel Company, 1931.
- **Gerber, Richard.** *Vibrational Medicine: The #1 Handbook of Subtle-Energy Therapies.* Rochester, VT: Bear & Co., 2001.
- **Kepner, James I.** *Body Process: A Gestalt Approach to Working with the Body in Psychotherapy.* San Francisco: Jossey-Bass, 1987.

About the Author

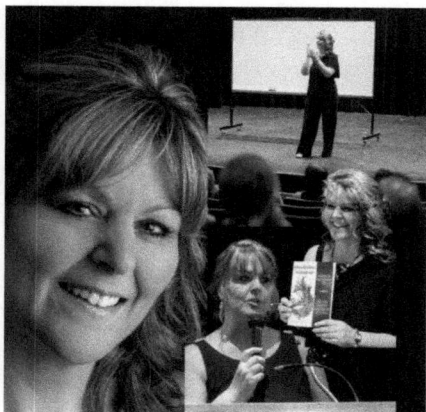

Dr. Constance Santego is a renowned educator, author, and expert in holistic health and spiritual healing. With over two decades of experience in teaching and clinical practice, she has guided thousands of students and clients in unlocking their innate healing potential.

Holding both a Ph.D. and a Doctorate in Natural Medicine, Dr. Santego bridges the wisdom of traditional healing with the insights of modern science. Her integrated approach to wellness reflects a deep understanding of how the mind, body, and spirit are intimately connected—and how imbalance in one area affects the whole.

As the creator of the *Secrets of a Healer* educational series, Dr. Santego shares the powerful techniques she has developed and refined over years of practice. Her books—each rooted in experience and energetic understanding—guide readers through the deeper language of healing, intuition, and energy medicine.

In *Signs and Meanings of the Feet*, Dr. Santego reveals the subtle stories told through the feet—stories that often precede words, symptoms, or diagnoses. Her ability to read the body's silent signals offers practitioners and wellness seekers a profound tool for early detection, intuitive healing, and deeper client connection.

Known for her warmth, clarity, and empowering style, Dr. Santego continues to inspire transformation through her writing, teachings, and personal healing philosophy:

"When we learn to listen to what the body shows, healing becomes inevitable."

MESSAGE FROM THE AUTHOR

Since 1997, I've had the privilege of working with countless feet—each pair telling its own unique story. Over time, I began to notice consistent patterns in markings, tension, texture, and pain that often corresponded with the client's physical, emotional, or energetic concerns—even when no diagnosis had yet been made. This book was born from those observations.

Signs and Meanings of the Feet is not meant to replace traditional reflexology or modern medicine. Rather, it complements both by offering a deeper layer of insight—an intuitive, pattern-based understanding of what the body silently reveals through the feet. Sometimes the signs show up before words can, or before tests confirm what a person already feels deep inside.

My goal in writing this guide is to empower you as a practitioner or curious learner to *look closer, listen deeper*, and *trust what you see and feel*—while always staying grounded in ethics, neutrality, and compassion. When we approach the body with respect, and our clients with presence, healing is no longer just a technique—it becomes a conversation.

Thank you for allowing me to share what I've learned on this journey. May it inspire your own path of discovery, and may you never look at a foot the same way again.

In wellness and wonder,
Dr. Constance Santego

Also by Dr. Constance Santego:
Secrets of a Healer – Magic of Reflexology

Used as the core manual in Dr. Santego's Reflexology Certification program, this book is more than a guide—it's a doorway into the healing power of the feet.

Magic of Reflexology blends science, energy work, and holistic awareness into one powerful learning experience. Designed for both students and practitioners, this book introduces the full-body reflexology map through detailed instruction, intuitive insight, and hands-on application.

Inside, you'll learn:

- How to apply precise techniques that stimulate reflex zones in the feet
- How reflexology supports circulation, stress reduction, and system balance
- How to use energy awareness and observation to enhance each session
- How to practice ethically and effectively in a wellness or clinical setting

Infused with real teaching examples and stories from the treatment room, *Magic of Reflexology* equips learners with the skills and confidence to become professional reflexologists—or to simply help others through the healing language of touch.

This foundational book laid the groundwork for the next volume, *Signs and Meanings*, which takes foot interpretation to a deeper level—before the session even begins.

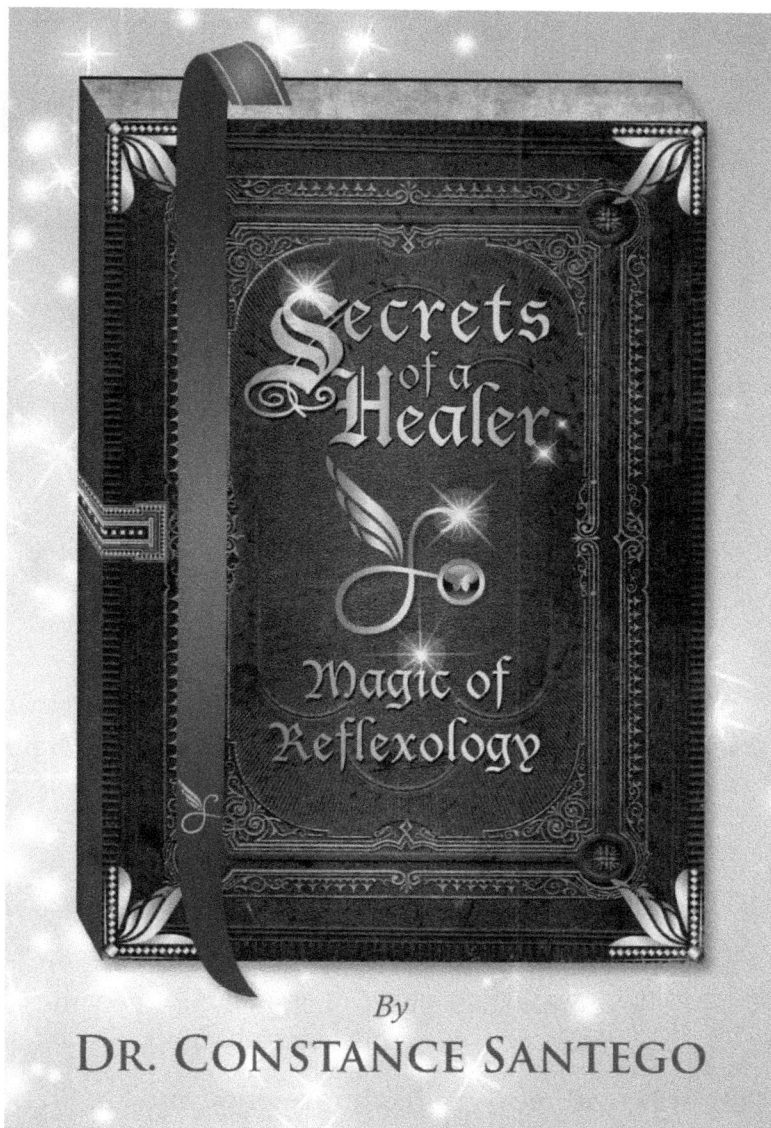

By
DR. CONSTANCE SANTEGO

Trade paperback ISBN: 978-1-989013-01-4
eBook ISBN 978-1-989013-09-0

Play the game *Ikona* – Discover Your Inner Genie

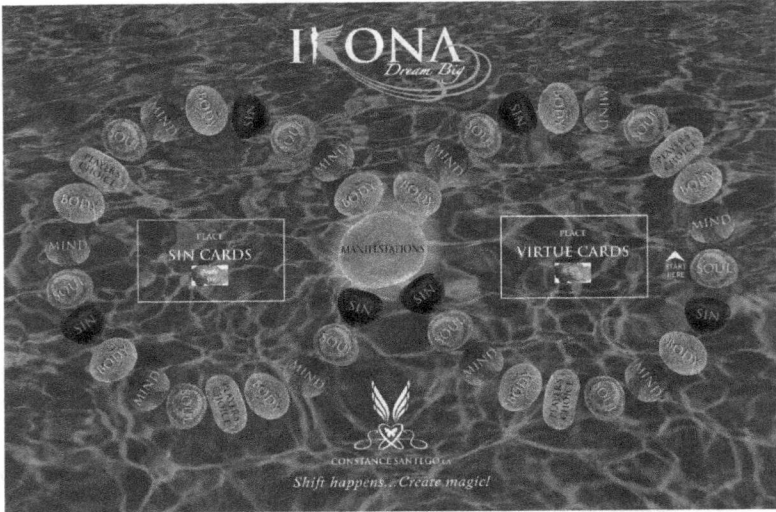

For additional information on

Constance Santego's

wide range of Motivational Products, Coaching Sessions,
Spiritual Retreats,
Live Events and Educational Programs

Go to

www.ConstanceSantego.ca

Follow on Instagram - Constance_Santego and
Facebook - constancesantegoo

Subscribe and receive Free Information and Meditations
on my
YouTube Channel - Constance Santego

DR. CONSTANCE SANTEGO

DR. CONSTANCE SANTEGO